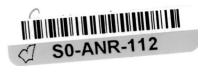

Kinesiological Bases for Exercise and Sport

Revised Printing

Danny Too
SUNY—Brockport

Christopher D. Williams
SUNY—Brockport

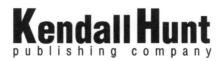

Kendall Hunt
publishing company

Exam 1

10 - What is kinesiology, biomechanics, statics, dynamics, kinetics, kinematics

10 - Planes + axis

9 - joint movement terminology

7 - movement instructions

8 - movement / skill analysis

9 - roles of muscles / types of contractions

Illustrations by Jamey Garbett © 2003 Mark Nielsen

Kendall Hunt
publishing company

www.kendallhunt.com
Send all inquiries to:
4050 Westmark Drive
Dubuque, IA 52004-1840

Revised Printing: 2011

ISBN 978-0-7575-8749-8

Printed in the United States of America
20 19 18 17 16 15 14 13

Contents

Introduction

Kinesiology

What Is Kinesiology?

1. Kinesiology is the study of movement (i.e., mammals, reptiles, fishes, birds, insects, invertebrates, etc.).
2. In Kinesiological/Exercise/Movement Science and Physical Education, kinesiology is concerned with the scientific study of human movement in sports, exercise, dance, and adaptive activities from different perspectives (e.g., mechanical, physiological, psychological, philosophical, historical, sociological, sports medicine, etc.).
3. In Structural or Anatomical Kinesiology, emphasis is on the study of bones, joints, and muscles involved in human movement.
4. In Mechanical Kinesiology (or Biomechanics), emphasis is on the study of forces and space and time factors involved in human movement using principles and concepts in mechanical physics.

In Physical Education, Kinesiology is often the name of a course used to study the anatomical basis of human movement which may or may not include the application of mechanical principles.

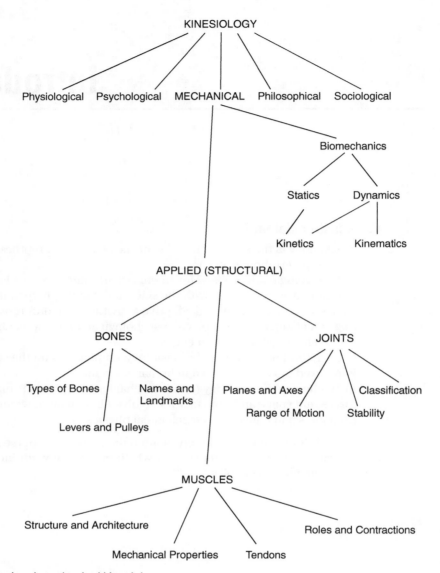

Figure I   Anatomical and mechanical kinesiology.

Why Study Kinesiology?

1. To learn how to analyze human movement and to discover the underlying principles of movement
2. To improve performance by modifying movement patterns with respect to normal movements (when recovering from injury, or using a prosthesis) or with respect to that of an elite athlete
3. To increase the safety, effectiveness, and efficiency of movement

The purpose of this book is to present an anatomical foundation for the analysis of human movement and how muscle forces involved in facilitating or inhibiting movement are modified.

The first part of the book will deal with anatomical structures, reference frames involved in movement, movement terminology, and worksheets for analyzing movements. Chapter 1 will examine the bones that comprise the axial and appendicular skeleton and the various anatomical landmarks where muscles attach. Chapter 2 will present the segmental reference frames used to describe and analyze movements, along with a description of different joint movements using scientific terminology. This will include a series of progressions and worksheets that have been designed to facilitate an understanding of joint movements in different planes and axes, and an introduction in analyzing selected movements and skills

The second part of this book will examine muscles of the axial and appendicular skeleton, their attachments (origins and insertions), roles, and actions possible at single and multiple joints. Chapter 3 will examine muscles of the trunk and neck. Chapters 4 through 7 will examine muscles of the upper extremities (scapula, humerus, forearm, wrist, hand, fingers, thumb), whereas Chapters 8 and 9 will cover the muscles of the lower extremites (hip, femur, leg, ankle, foot). The chapters and accompanying worksheets have been designed to facilitate learning of not just all the joint actions possible by individual muscles, but also with any given joint action, what are all the muscles and muscle groups involved.

The third part of this book will discuss how movements are analyzed, how a skill can be broken down into phases and sub-phases, how muscles are recruited to produce the desired movement or joint action, and how muscle forces can be modified to affect movement and skill activities. Chapter 10 examines a series of progressions used to analyze a skill and how to determine the muscle groups and contraction involved. Chapter 11 will discuss the roles of muscles as neutralizers and stabilizers and how various combinations of muscles might be recruited to produce the desired joint action yet neutralize other unwanted actions or movements. Chapter 12 will present a mechanical analysis of the skeletal system. This chapter on skeletal mechanics will include information regarding how muscle torque is modified by a combination of levers, pulleys, and wheel and axle interacting to affect the resultant force and torque produced. This will involve a discussion of the different levers and pulleys found in the body, as well as how these have been incorporated into resistance training machines. This will also include information regarding the use of cams in resistance training machines and how different combinations of levers, pulleys, and cams modify the resistance that needs to be lifted. Chapter 13 will present a mechanical analysis of the muscular system. This will include information regarding muscle mechanics, how muscle forces are altered by changes in muscle length, velocity of contraction, type of contraction, fiber type, and architecture. Information will also be presented regarding the musculotendinous unit and contribution to total muscle tension (active and passive) by its various components. In addition, information will be presented in regards to strength curves and how muscle force and torque are modified by an interaction of skeletal mechanics with muscle mechanics.

PART I

Foundations of
Anatomical Kinesiology

Objectives

To be able to:
1. identify the different bones in the axial and appendicular skeleton
2. determine the number of bones for different parts of the axial and appendicular skeleton
3. locate and identify the anatomical landmarks for different bones
4. determine the orientation and perspective of different bones
5. classify joints according to function

The Skeletal System

Purpose:
1. To protect internal organs
2. To provide rigid kinematic links
3. To provide muscle attachment sites
4. To provide a lever system to permit movement
5. To contain marrow which manufactures blood cells

Facts:
1. Bone is one of the most dynamic and metabolically active tissues of the body.
2. Bone is highly vascular with an excellent capacity for self-repair and can alter its property and configuration in response to changes in mechanical demand.
3. Bone has a high content of inorganic materials, in the form of mineral salts (calcium and phosphate), that combine with an organic matrix.
4. The inorganic mineral salts make bone hard and rigid (~65–70%).
5. The organic component makes bone flexible and resilient (~5%).
6. Water accounts for ~25%.

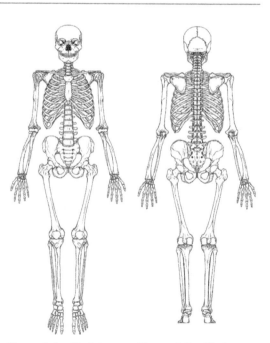

Figure 1.1 Skeleton, anterior view.

Figure 1.2 Skeleton, posterior view.

Types of Bone Tissue:
1. Cortical Bone (Compact)—dense structure that forms the cortex of a bone (outer shell).
2. Cancellous Bone (Trabecular)—loose, mesh structure filled with red marrow, surrounded by the cortex.

Types of Bone:
1. Long—cylindrical shaft, central cavity (humerus, radius, ulna, femur, tibia, fibula, metacarpals, metatarsals, phalanges)
2. Short—small, solid (carpals and tarsals)
3. Flat (sternum, scapula, ribs, ilium, patella)
4. Irregular (vertebrae, ischium, pubis, maxilla)
5. Sesamoid (patella, hyoid, bones of the ear)

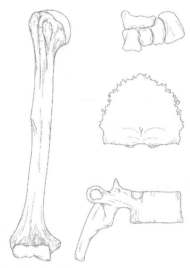

Figure 1.3   Types of bones.

Mechanical Axis of a Bone
The mechanical axis of a bone or segment is a straight line that connects the midpoint of the joint at the one end with the midpoint of the joint at the other end (or the distal end).

Total number of bones at birth is <u>270–300</u>. The adult skeleton contains <u>206</u> bones. This does not include wormian bones (bones between sutures of the skull) or sesamoids (floating bones) other than the patella (kneecap).

The bones of the body are divided into two groups, the <u>axial</u> skeleton and the <u>appendicular</u> skeleton.

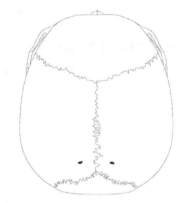

Figure 1.4   Cranium, superior view.

Adult Axial Skeleton (80 total bones)

1. Skull   29 bones

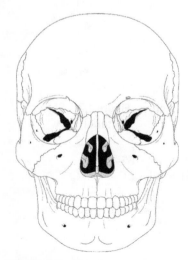

Figure 1.5   Cranium, anterior view.

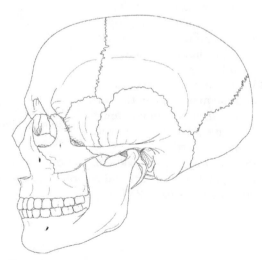

Figure 1.6   Cranium, lateral view.

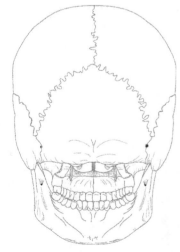

Figure 1.7   Cranium, posterior view.

2. Vertebral column   26 bones

7 cervical vertebrae
12 thoracic vertebrae
5 lumbar vertebrae
1 sacrum (5 fused bones)
1 coccyx (4 fused bones)

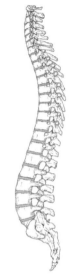

Figure 1.8   Vertebral column, lateral view.

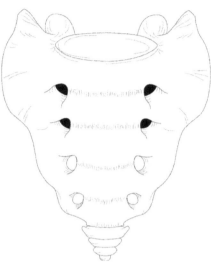

Figure 1.9   Sacrum, anterior view.

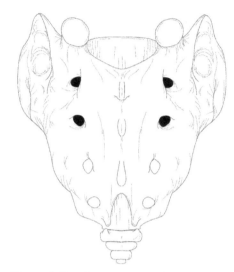

Figure 1.10   Sacrum, posterior view.

The first cervical vertebrae is called the <u>atlas vertebra</u>.

The second cervical vertebrae is called the <u>axis vertebra</u>.

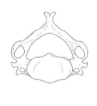

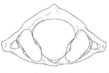

Figure 1.11   Cervical vertebrae, superior view.

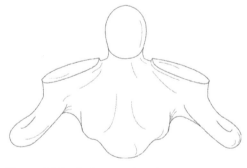

Figure 1.12   Axis, anterior view.

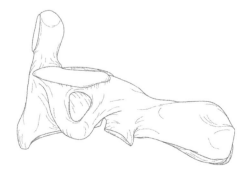

Figure 1.13   Axis, lateral view.

There are 26 bones in the vertebral column with 24 vertebra.

Vertebrae
   a. C1—atlas
   b. C2—axis (dens process)
   c. body
   d. vertebral foramen
   e. spinous process
   f. superior/inferior articular surface
   g. superior/inferior costal surface
   h. transverse process

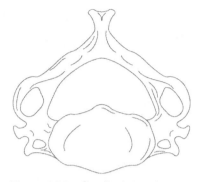

Figure 1.14   Cervical vertebra, superior view.

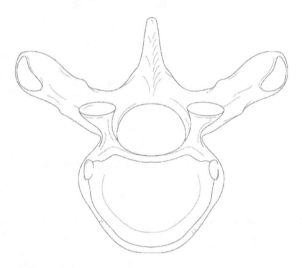

Figure 1.15   Thoracic vertebra, superior view.

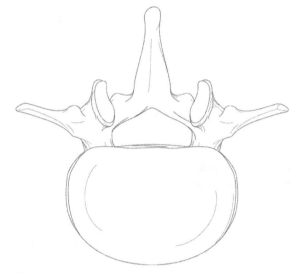

Figure 1.16   Lumbar vertebra, superior view.

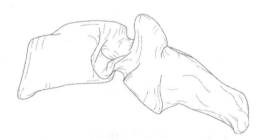

Figure 1.17   Cervical vertebra, lateral view.

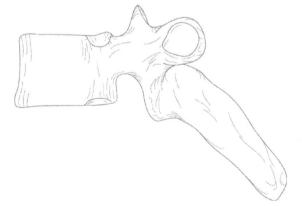

Figure 1.18   Thoracic vertebra, lateral view.

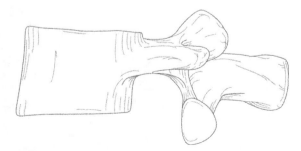

Figure 1.19   Lumbar vertebra, lateral view.

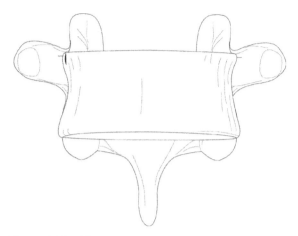

Figure 1.20   Thoracic vertebra, anterior view.

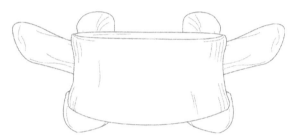

Figure 1.21   Lumbar vertebra, anterior view.

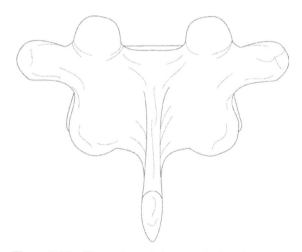

Figure 1.22   Thoracic vertebra, posterior view.

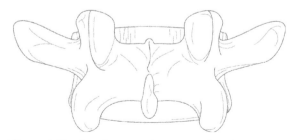

Figure 1.23   Lumbar vertebra, posterior view.

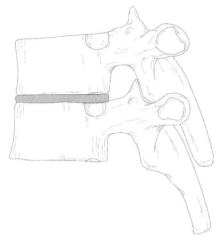

Figure 1.24   Thoracic vertebrae articulated.

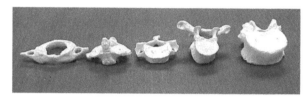

Figure 1.25   Atlas, axis, cervical, thoracic, lumbar vertebrae (anterior view).

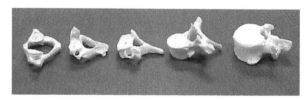

Figure 1.26   Atlas, axis, cervical, thoracic, lumbar vertebrae (lateral view).

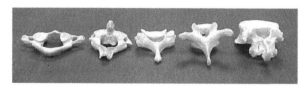

Figure 1.27   Atlas, axis, cervical, thoracic, lumbar vertebrae (posterior view).

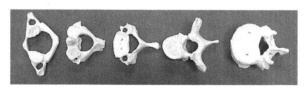

Figure 1.28   Atlas, axis, cervical, thoracic, lumbar vertebrae (superior view).

3. Thorax   25 bones   1 sternum

                                                 manubrium
                                                 body
                                                 xiphoid process

                        24 ribs (12 pairs of ribs)

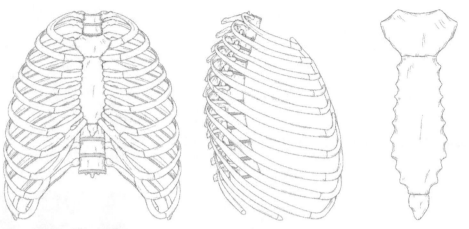

Figure 1.29 Thoracic cage, anterior view.

Figure 1.30 Thoracic cage, lateral view.

Figure 1.31 Sternum, anterior view.

The first 7 pairs of ribs are called true ribs.

The last 5 pairs of ribs are called ____false____ ribs.

The last 2 pairs of false ribs are called ___floating___ ribs

Appendicular Skeleton

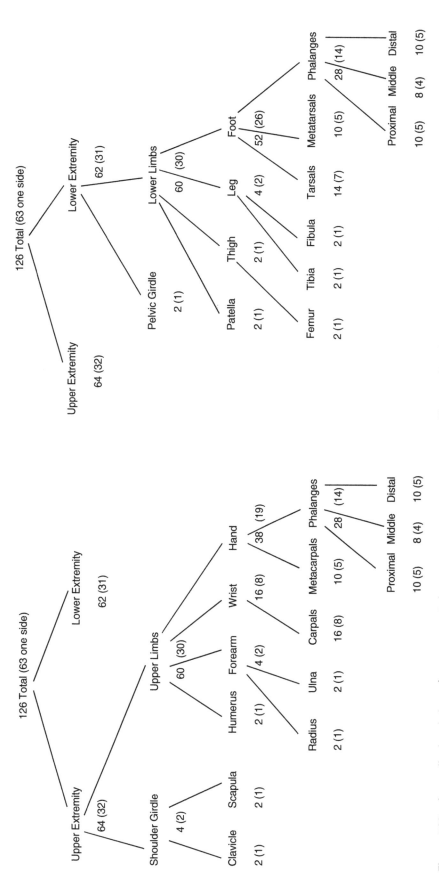

Figure 1.32 Appendicular skeleton (upper extremity).

Figure 1.33 Appendicular skeleton (lower extremity).

Table 1.1. Adult Appendicular Skeleton (126 total bones)

	Total				One Side			
1. Upper Extremities	**64**				**32**			
A. Shoulder Girdle	**4**				**2**			
i. Clavicle		2				1		
ii. Scapula		2				1		
B. Upper Limbs	**60**				**30**			
i. Humerus		2				1		
ii. Forearm		4				2		
a. Radius			2				1	
b. Ulna			2				1	
iii. Carpals		16				8		
iv. Hand		38				19		
a. Metacarpals			10				5	
b. Phalanges			28				14	
(i) Proximal				10				5
(ii) Middle				8				4
(iii) Distal				10				5
2. Lower Extremities	**62**				**31**			
A. Pelvic Girdle	**2**				**1**			
B. Lower Limbs	**60**				**30**			
i. Femur		2				1		
ii. Leg		4				2		
a. Tibia			2				1	
b. Fibula			2				1	
iii. Patella		2				1		
iv. Foot		52				26		
a. Tarsals			14				7	
b. Metatarsals			10				5	
c. Phalanges			28				14	
(i) Proximal				10				5
(ii) Middle				8				4
(iii) Distal				10				5

Upper Extremities

1. Clavicle (collar bone)

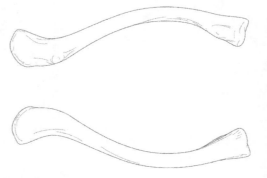

Figure 1.34   Clavicle.

2. Scapula
   a. supraspinous fossa
   b. infraspinous fossa
   c. subscapular fossa
   d. inferior angle
   e. superior angle
   f. spine of scapula (scapular spine)
   g. axillary border (lateral border)
   h. vertebral border (medial border)
   i. glenoid cavity
   j. acromion (acromion process)
   k. coracoid process

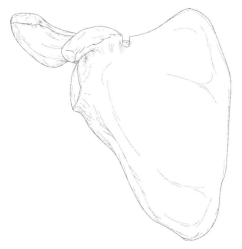

Figure 1.35   Scapula, anterior view.

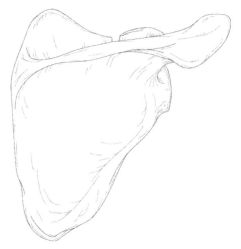

Figure 1.36   Scapula, posterior view.

3. Humerus
   a. head
   b. greater tubercle (tuberosity)
   c. lesser tubercle (tuberosity)
   d. intertubercular groove (bicipital groove)
   e. deltoid tuberosity
   f. lateral epicondyle
   g. medial epicondyle
   h. trochlea
   i. capitulum
   j. olecranon fossa
   k. coronoid fossa
4. Ulna
   a. coronoid process
   b. olecranon process
   c. semi-lunar notch
   d. radial notch
   e. styloid process of ulna

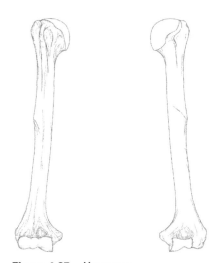

Figure 1.37   Humerus.

5. Radius
   a. head of radius
   b. radial tuberosity
   c. styloid process of radius

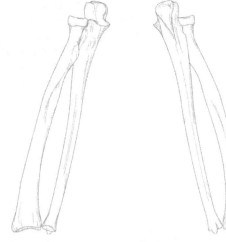

Figure 1.38 Radius and ulna, anterior view.   **Figure 1.39** Radius and ulna, posterior view.

6. Hand
   a. metacarpals (5)
   b. proximal phalanges (5)
   c. middle phalanges (4)
   d. distal phalanges (5)

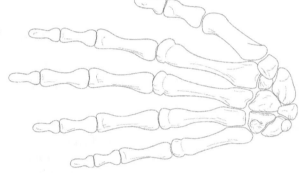

Figure 1.40 Hand, anterior view.

Lower Extremities

1. Pelvic Girdle (Hip Bone, Os Coxae, Inominate Bone)
   a. ilium
      i. iliac crest
      ii. iliac fossa
      iii. iliac spine (anterior/posterior, superior/inferior)
      iv. sciatic notch
   b. ischium
      i. ischial spine (spine of ischium)
      ii. ischial tuberosity
      iii. ramus of ishium
   c. pubis
      i. pubic crest
      ii. symphysis pubis
      iii. ramus of pubis (superior/descending/inferior)
      iv. pectineal line
   d. acetabulum
   f. obturator foramen

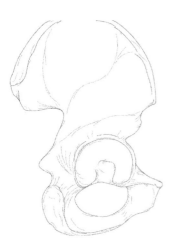

Figure 1.41 Os coxa, lateral view.

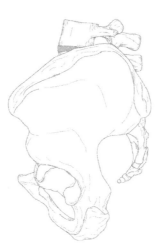

Figure 1.42 Female pelvis, lateral view.

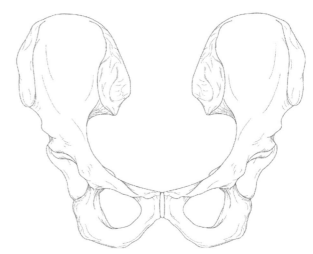

Figure 1.43 Os coxae articulated.

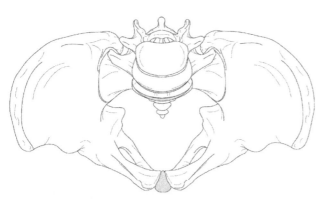

Figure 1.44 Male pelvis, superior view.

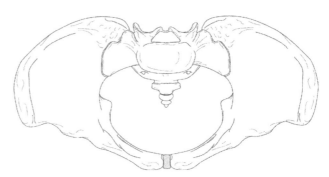

Figure 1.45 Female pelvis, superior view.

2. Femur
   a. head
   b. neck
   c. greater trochanter
   d. lesser trochanter
   e. intertrochanteric line
   f. intertrochanteric crest
   g. linea aspera
   h. epicondyles (medial, lateral)
   i. condyles (medial, lateral)
   j. intercondylar (patellar) groove
   k. intercondylar fossa
3. Tibia
   a. tibial plateau
   b. tibial tuberosity
   c. lateral condyle
   d. medial condyle
   e. intercondylar eminence
   f. medial malleolus

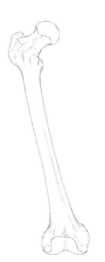

Figure 1.46 Femur, anterior view.

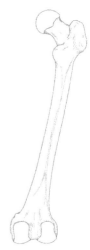

Figure 1.47 Femur, posterior view.

4. Fibula
   a. head
   b. lateral malleolus

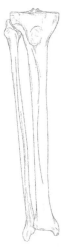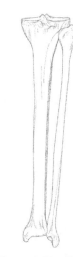

Figure 1.48 Tibia and fibula, anterior view.

Figure 1.49 Tibia and fibula, posterior view.

5. Patella (kneecap)

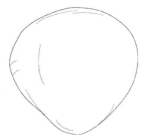

Figure 1.50 Patella, anterior view.

6. Foot
   a. 7 tarsals (calcaneus, talus, cuneiforms , [medial, intermediate, lateral], cuboid, navicular)
   b. 5 metatarsals
   c. 14 phalanges (5 proximal, 4 middle, 5 distal)

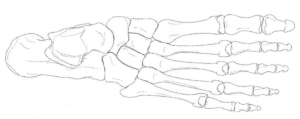

Figure 1.51 Foot, superior view.

Note: 14 total segments that can form a kinematic chain (head, trunk, shoulder girdle, humerus, ulna, radius, wrist, hand, pelvic girdle, femur, tibia, fibula, ankle, foot)

Kinematic Chain
1. A series of successive (adjoined, articulating) segments
2. A series of single joint systems

Joints

Functional (Structural) Classification

I. Synarthrotic (Fibrous)—no movement
1. Edges of the bones are united by a thin layer of fibrous tissue.
2. Examples: sutures of the skull, sockets of the teeth

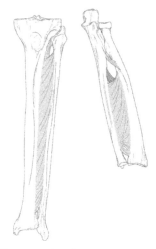

Figure 1.52   Syndesmoses—interosseous membranes.

II. Amphiarthrotic (Cartilaginous)—slightly movable
1. Bones are connected/separated by ligaments, fibrocartilage, or hyaline cartilage that allows very slight movement between the bones.
2. Examples: coracoclavicular joint, tibiofibular joint, symphysis pubis, intervertebral discs, costochondral joints of the ribs with the sternum
III. Diarthrotic (synovial)—movable
A. Characteristics
1. An articular cavity is present.
2. The joint is encased within a ligamentous sheath called the synovial capsule.
3. The capsule is lined with the synovial membrane that secretes synovial fluid for lubrication.
4. The articular surfaces of the bones are covered with hyaline cartilage and occasionally fibrocartilage.
B. Classification
1. Irregular
a. Joint surfaces are irregularly shaped, usually flat or slightly curved
b. Planar movement only
c. Nonaxial
d. Movement is of a gliding nature
e. Examples: carpal joints, tarsal joints

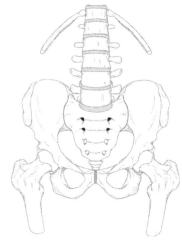

Figure 1.53   Cartilaginous joints—symphyses.

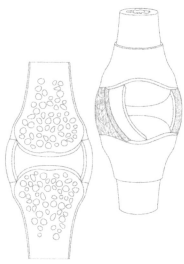

Figure 1.54   Diarthrotic joint.

2. Hinge
   a. A concave surface rotates around a convex protuberance
   b. Movement in one plane about a single axis
   c. Uniaxial (one rotational degree of freedom)
   d. Movement is flexion and extension
   e. Examples: elbow joint, knee joint

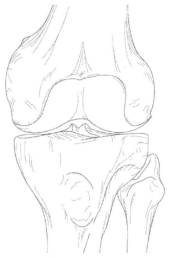

Figure 1.55   Knee joint, anterior view.

3. Pivot
   a. Characterized by a peg-like pivot, or as a long bone rolls about another one on the long axis of the bones
   b. Movement in one plane about a single axis
   c. Uniaxial (one rotational degree of freedom)
   d. Movement is rotation
   e. Examples: atlas-axis joint, radio-ulnar joint

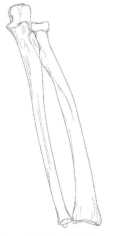

Figure 1.56   Radio-ulnar joints.

4. Condyloid
   a. Joint surfaces are concave and convex
   b. Movement can occur in two planes and two axes
   c. Biaxial (two rotational degrees of freedom)
   d. Movement is flexion/extension, abduction/adduction, and circumduction
   e. Examples: wrist joint (radio-carpal, unlar-carpal), metacarpo-phalangeal joints, ankle joint, metatarsal-phalangeal joints

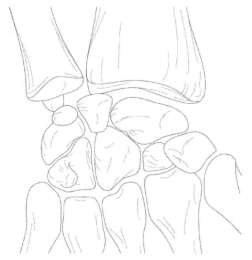

Figure 1.57   Wrist joint.

5. Saddle
   a. Joint surfaces are concave-convex
   b. Movement can occur in two planes and two axes
   c. Biaxial (two rotational degrees of freedom)
   d. Movement is flexion/extension, abduction/adduction, and circumduction
   e. Can be considered a modified condyloid joint with greater range of motion
   f. Examples: thumb (carpo-metacarpal joint)
6. Ball-and-Socket Joint
   a. A spherical protuberance (head of bone) is fitted into a cup-shaped (concave) cavity
   b. Movement can occur in three planes and three axes
   c. Triaxial (three rotational degrees of freedom)
   d. Movement is flexion/extension, abduction/adduction, circumduction, horizontal abduction/adduction, and rotation
   e. Examples: hip, shoulder

Summary

Table 1.2. Degrees of Freedom for Different Joint Classification					
Number of Planes	0	1	1	2	3
Number of Axes	0	0	1	2	3
Classification	Fibrous	Irregular	Hinge Pivot	Condyloid Saddle	Ball-Socket Cartilaginous

Joint Stability and Range of Motion

The function of the joints is to provide the bones with a means of being moved (by muscles).

As a joint becomes more "movable," it loses stability. For example, movement is gained at the shoulder at the expense of stability; whereas, stability is gained at the hip at the expense of movement (range of motion).

Based on the strength and stability at a joint, the potential for injury can be determined (e.g., the shoulder vs. the hip, the knee vs. the elbow).

A. Factors of Joint Stability—resistance to displacement
   1. The shape of the bony structure.
      a. Specific characteristics of a joint can lead to different levels of stability (e.g., shoulder vs. hip).
   2. Ligaments
      a. Ligaments are strong, flexible, fibrous tissues that connect bone to bone and inhibit motion when stretched.
      b. Ligaments restrict joint movement to a specific range of motion (normal limits) (e.g., the ligaments of the knee).
      c. Due to a lack of elasticity, ligaments do not return quickly to their normal length when stretched.
      d. If overstretched, ligaments can deform or tear such that normal length is never regained and joint stability is permanently compromised.

   3. Muscles
      a. Muscular structure can affect joint stability, especially at joints that are inherently unstable (e.g., the shoulder or knee).
      b. Muscles, acting as stabilizers (discussed later), are used as an important joint stabilizer by increasing muscular strength, especially when ligaments have been injured.
      c. Muscular strength of the muscles crossing a joint is the dominant factor affecting joint stability (see Factors Affecting Range of Motion that follows).
   4. Fascia and Skin
      a. Fascia is a non-elastic, fibrous tissue that varies in structure from thin membranes to thick sheets.
      b. Like ligaments, fascia is susceptible to stretch.
      c. Fascia and skin surround joints and can help in stabilization to a limited extent.
   5. Atmospheric Pressure
      a. It has been experimentally shown that less pressure exists within the joint capsule of the hip such that a suction effect is created that pulls the head of the femur into the acetabulum and increases joint stability.
B. Factors Affecting Range of Motion
   1. The shape of the bony structure.
      a. Often, the bony structure will physically limit ROM (e.g., the elbow).
   2. Ligaments
      a. As previously stated, ligaments connect bone to bone, are resistant to stretch, and will inhibit motion when stretched.
   3. Muscles
      a. Muscles are very elastic and will readily return to their original shape when stretched.
      b. The degree of stretch possible is affected by repeatedly moving to the limits of one's ROM.
      c. In addition, the degree of stretch is moderated by proprioceptive function of muscle spindles and Golgi Tendon organs (discussed later).
      d. The size of a muscle may also limit movement (i.e., bodybuilders).
   4. Body Build
      a. Ectomorphs and mesomorphs are generally more flexible than endomorphs.
      b. Any bulky tissue can affect ROM.
   5. Gender
      a. Generally, females are more flexible than males due to hormonal differences that can affect the laxity of ligaments and tendons.
   6. Heredity
      a. Bony structure, body build, and muscular arrangement are genetically determined.
   7. Level of Fitness and Exercise Habits
      a. People with higher levels of fitness and consistent patterns of exercise have greater ROM and greater muscular strengths.

There is a close relationship between range of motion, joint stability, and risk of injury. Generally, muscle function is the dominant factor that will determine the difference between normal joint function and injury for any given movement.

WORKSHEET 1.1

Skeleton

1. For the pictures of bones of the axial skeleton, identify the
   a. bone
   b. view (superior, inferior, anterior, posterior, medial, lateral, etc.)
   c. orientation (right side up, up side down, side ways)
   d. anatomical landmarks (as presented in class)
   Depending on the view, identify (where appropriate) the superior, inferior, medial, and lateral side of the bone.
2. For pictures of bones of the appendicular skeleton, identify the
   a. bone
   b. side (right or left)
   c. view (superior, inferior, anterior, posterior, medial, lateral)
   d. orientation (right side up, up side down, side ways)
   e. anatomical landmarks (as presented in class)
   Depending on the view, identify (where appropriate) the superior, inferior, medial, lateral, anterior, and posterior side of the bone.

Axial Skeleton

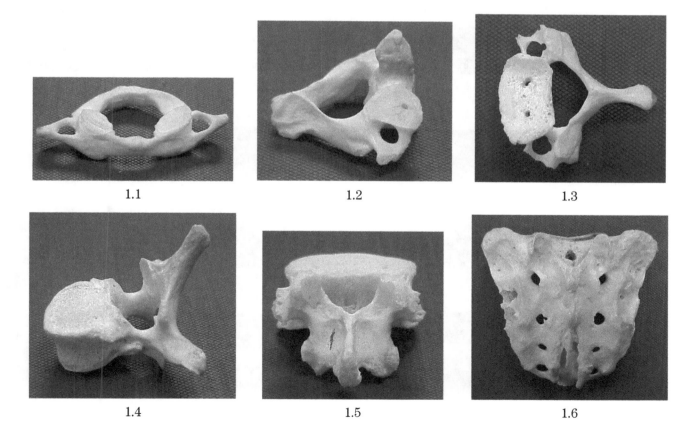

1.1

1.2

1.3

1.4

1.5

1.6

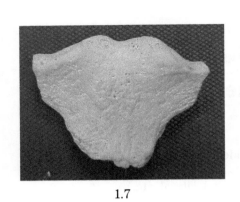

1.7

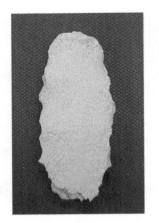

1.8

Appendicular Skeleton

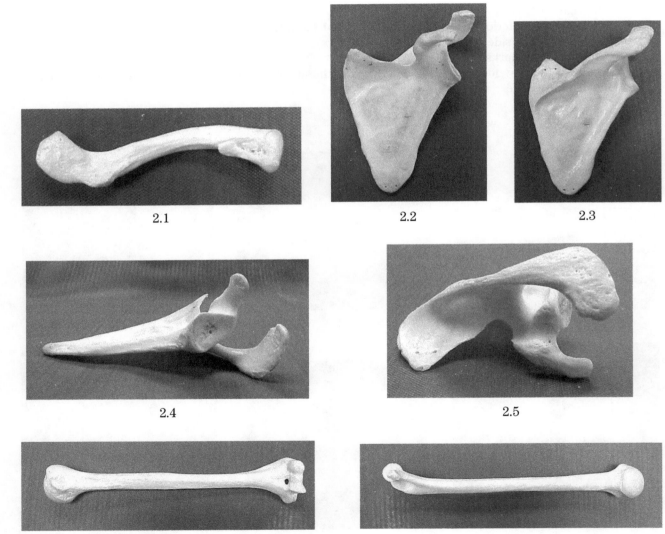

2.1

2.2

2.3

2.4

2.5

2.6

2.7

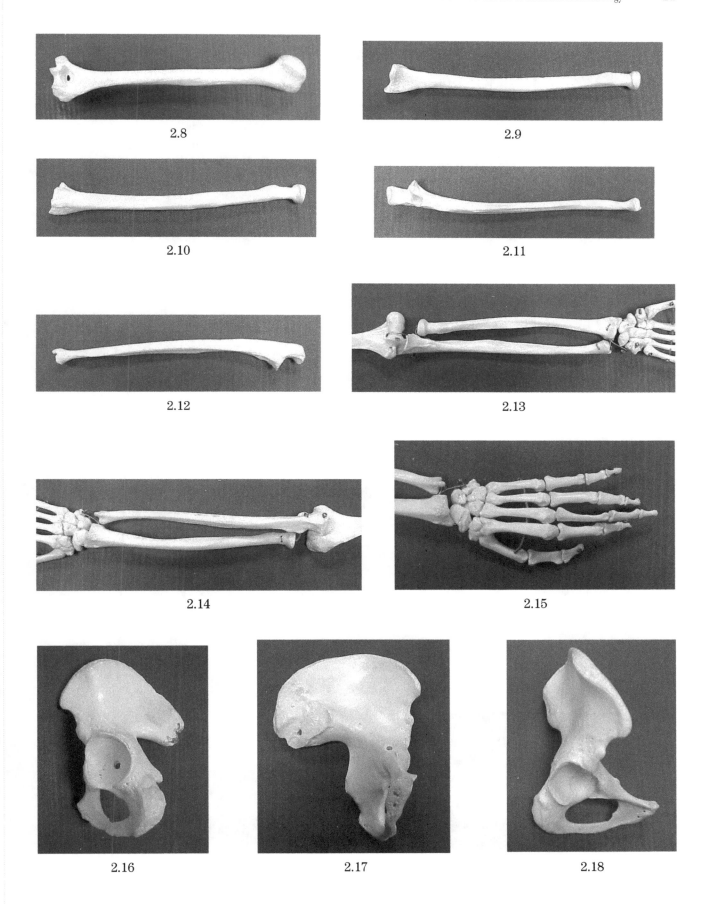

2.8

2.9

2.10

2.11

2.12

2.13

2.14

2.15

2.16

2.17

2.18

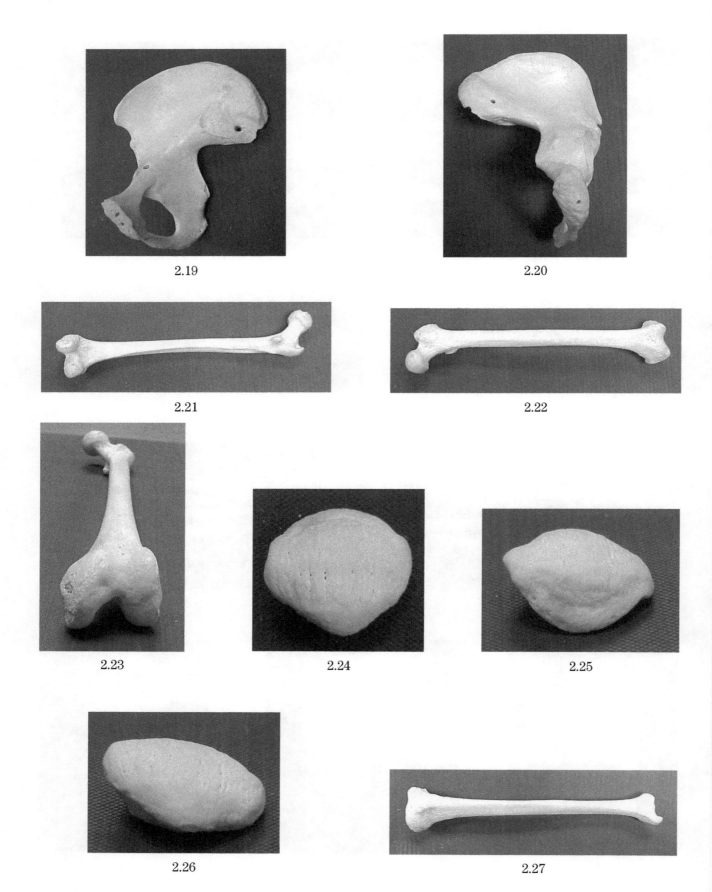

2.19

2.20

2.21

2.22

2.23

2.24

2.25

2.26

2.27

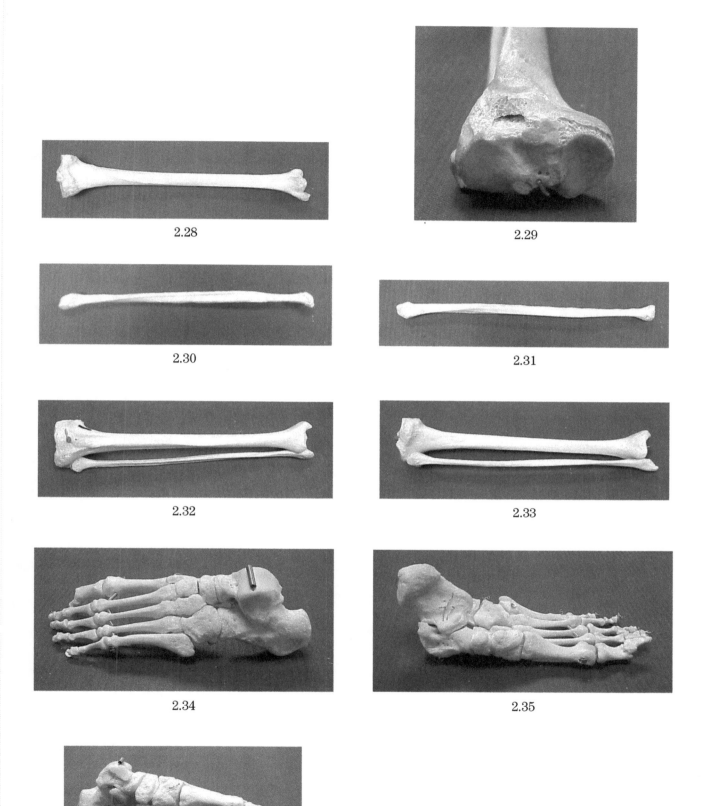

2.28

2.29

2.30

2.31

2.32

2.33

2.34

2.35

2.36

CHAPTER 2

Planes and Axes and Movement Terminology

Objectives

To be able to:

1. name the planes and axes of motion of the body
2. provide examples of movement activities that occur in different planes and axes
3. identify and demonstrate all possible joint actions in the different planes and axes
4. follow movement instructions given in scientific terminology and identify the plane and axis of different joint movements
5. give movement instructions in scientific terminology with corresponding planes and axes
6. break a skill or movement activity into phases, and for each phase identify all the joint actions and corresponding planes and axes of motion

Human Anatomy Terminology

1. Regions of the Body
   a. antibrachial—forearm
   b. axilla—armpit
   c. brachial—upper arm
   d. calcaneal—heel
   e. carpal—wrist
   f. cervical—neck
   g. cubital—elbow
   h. femoral—thigh
   i. hallux—big toe
   j. lumbar—lower back
   k. metacarpal—hand
   l. metatarsal—foot
   m. nuchae—back of neck
   n. pectoral—chest
   o. peroneal—lower leg (lateral side)
   p. plantar—sole of foot
   q. pollex—thumb
   r. popliteal—back of knee
   s. tarsal—ankle
   t. thoracic—chest
   u. volar—palm of hand
2. Anatomical Directions
   a. distal—away from the center of mass of the body
   b. proximal—nearer to the center of mass of the body
   c. superior (cranial)—above (closer to the head)
   d. inferior (caudal)—below (further from the head)

   e. deep (central)—away from the surface
   f. superficial (peripheral)—nearer to the surface
   g. dorsal—the back of a body part (hand, foot, back)
   h. palmar—palm of the hand
   i. plantar—bottom of the foot
   j. anterior (ventral)—towards the front
   k. posterior (dorsal)—towards the back
   l. medial—toward the midline of the body
   m. lateral—away from the midline of the body
3. Bony Markings
   a. condyle—a large, smooth, rounded prominence
   b. epicondyle—a small, smooth, rounded prominence
   c. line—a long narrow ridge
   d. spine—a sharp projection
   e. crest—a ridge
   f. stylus—a pencil-point projection
   g. tubercle, tuberosity, trochanter—an eminence or enlargement
   h. fossa—a depression or hollow
   i. foramen—a hole through a bone
   j. head—a smooth rounded end of a bone
   k. neck—a constriction below the head of a bone
4. Other terms
   a. longitudinal axis—the long axis of a bone or segment
   b. cross-sectional axis—the short axis of a bone or segment that is perpendicular to the long axis

Planes and Axes That Define Human Motion

Orientation of the Body

Line of Gravity—an imaginary vertical line that passes through the center of gravity of an object and represents the pull of gravity on the object.

Plane—an imaginary surface such that all points on a straight line lie on the surface. A plane has only two dimensions and is, therefore, infinitely thin.

Axis—an imaginary line about which a body rotates. An axis is always perpendicular to a plane (and has only one dimension).

Cardinal (Principle) Plane or Axis—a plane or axis that passes through the center of gravity and divides the body symmetrically.

When describing human motion, the reference position is always assumed to be either the anatomical or fundamental position.

Anatomical Position—the body is standing upright with the arms at the sides and the palms turned forward.

Figure 2.1 Planes and sections.

Fundamental Position—the body is standing upright with the arms at the sides and the palms facing the body.

Planes

1. Sagittal (also Median, Antero-Posterior)—a vertical plane passing through the body from front to back and dividing the body into right and left sections.
2. Frontal (also Medio-Lateral, Coronal)—a vertical plane passing through the body from left to right and dividing the body into anterior and posterior sections.
3. Transverse (also Horizontal)—a horizontal plane passing through the body (front to back and right to left) and dividing the body into superior and inferior sections.
4. Diagonal (also Oblique)—any plane that does not fit into any of the previous definitions.

circumduction

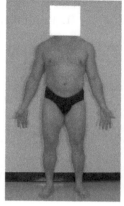

Figure 2.2
Anatomical position.

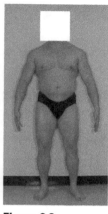

Figure 2.3
Fundamental position.

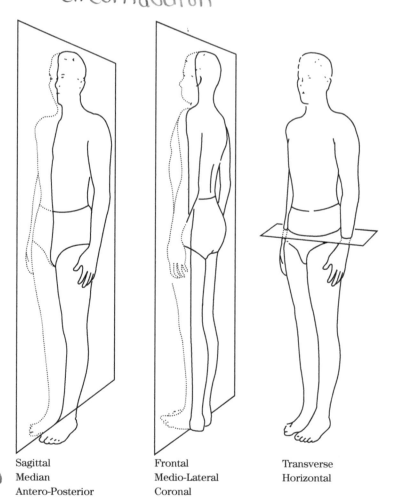

Sagittal	Frontal	Transverse
Median	Medio-Lateral	Horizontal
Antero-Posterior	Coronal	

(Sam)

Figure 2.4   Planes of Motion.

Axes

1. Frontal-Horizontal (also Medio-Lateral, Frontal-Transverse, Bilateral)—
   a horizontal axis that is perpendicular to the sagittal plane and passes through
   the body from one side to the other side.
2. Sagittal-Horizontal (also Antero-Posterior, Sagittal-Transverse)—a horizontal
   axis that is perpendicular to the frontal plane and passes through the body
   from anterior to posterior.
3. Sagittal-Frontal (also Vertical, Longitudinal, Polar)—a vertical axis that is
   perpendicular to the transverse plane and passes through the body from
   superior to inferior.
4. Diagonal (Oblique)—any axis that does not fit into any of the previous
   definitions.

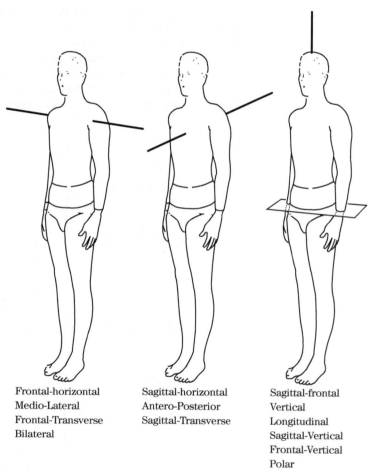

Frontal-horizontal	Sagittal-horizontal	Sagittal-frontal
Medio-Lateral	Antero-Posterior	Vertical
Frontal-Transverse	Sagittal-Transverse	Longitudinal
Bilateral		Sagittal-Vertical
		Frontal-Vertical
		Polar

Figure 2.5   Axes of Motion.

Examples of activities in the

Sagittal Plane: bowling, walking, somersault, chopping wood, front crawl in
swimming, volleyball overhead serve, front splits

Frontal Plane: jumping jacks, cartwheel, elementary backstroke, roundhouse
serve in volleyball, side splits

Transverse Plane: baseball swing, tennis forehand/backhand, discus throw,
karate roundhouse kick, hammer throw

Movement Terminology (from Anatomical Position)

Sagittal Plane

1. flexion—a decrease in joint angle (neck, trunk, shoulder, elbow, wrist, hand/fingers, hip, knee, ankle, foot/toes)
2. extension—an increase in joint angle
3. hyperflexion—flexion of a joint such that the joint angle is less than 0 degrees (negatively increasing)
4. hyperextension—extension of a joint such that the joint angle exceeds 180 degrees
5. upward tilt—movement of the inferior angle of the scapula posteriorly (away from the ribs)
6. downward tilt—movement of the inferior angle of the scapula anteriorly (toward from the ribs)
7. anterior pelvic tilt or rotation—forward tilt of upper pelvis (iliac crest)
8. posterior pelvic tilt or rotation—backward tilt of upper pelvis (iliac crest)
9. plantar flexion—movement of the foot downward (pointing your toes) (also called extension)
10. dorsal flexion—movement of the foot upward, toward the anterior surface of the leg (also called flexion)

Frontal Plane

1. abduction—movement away from the midline of the body (neck, trunk, shoulder, wrist, metacarpophalangeal joint, hip, ankle)
2. adduction—movement toward the midline of the body
3. hyperabduction—abduction of a joint (usually shoulder) more than 180 degrees
4. hyperadduction—adduction of joint (usually shoulder or hip) past the midline of the body
5. lateral flexion (right or left)—movement of the neck or trunk to the side away from the midline of the body
6. reduction—return from lateral flexion
7. elevation—movement that raises the scapula
8. depression—movement that lowers the scapula
9. upward rotation—rotation of the scapula such that the inferior angle moves upward (laterally)
10. downward rotation—rotation of the scapula such that the inferior angle moves downward (medially)
11. radial flexion or radial deviation—movement of the thumb side of the hand towards the radius
12. ulnar flexion or ulnar deviation—movement of the little finger side of the hand towards the ulna
13. lateral pelvic tilt or rotation (right or left)—right tilt occurs when right pelvis moves inferiorly to left pelvis
14. inversion—movement of the plantar side of the foot toward the midline of the body (refers to ankle)
15. eversion—movement of the plantar side of the foot away from the midline of the body (refers to ankle)

Transverse Plane

1. transverse, horizontal, or spinal rotation (left or right)—rotation of a segment that lies on the midline of the body (refers to neck and trunk)
2. protraction—anterior rotation of the scapula (away from the midline of the body)
3. retraction—posterior rotation of the scapula (towards the midline of the body)
4. lateral tilt—posterior movement of medial border of scapula and anterior movement of lateral border of scapula as a result of protraction

5. medial tilt—anterior movement of medial border of scapula and posterior movement of lateral border of scapula as a result of retraction from a protracted position (also, return from lateral tilt)
6. medial rotation—rotation of a segment about its longitudinal axis toward the midline of the body (refers to shoulder and hip)
7. lateral rotation—rotation of a segment about its longitudinal axis away from the midline of the body (refers to shoulder and hip)
8. horizontal flexion (horizontal adduction)—flexion in the transverse plane (refers to shoulder and hip and cannot be performed from anatomical position)
9. horizontal extension (horizontal abduction)—extension in the transverse plane (refers to shoulder and hip and cannot be performed from anatomical position)
10. pronation—rotation of the radio-ulnar joint toward the midline
11. supination—rotation of the radio-ulnar joint away from the midline

Other Terms

1. circumduction—a combination of flexion/extension and adduction/abduction (the segment forms the pattern of a cone) performed by the neck, trunk, shoulder, wrist, metacarpophalangeal joint, hip, ankle, and metatarsophalangeal joint.
2. diagonal abduction—movement of the humerus (or hip) in a diagonal plane away from the midline of the body
3. diagonal adduction—movement of the humerus (or hip) in a diagonal plane toward the midline of the body
4. foot pronation—combination of forefoot abduction, subtalar eversion, and ankle dorsiflexion
5. foot supination—combination of forefoot adduction, subtalar inversion, and ankle plantar flexion

Possible Joint Movements (from Anatomical Position)

Neck and Trunk

1. flexion/extension *sagittal*
2. hyperextension
3. a. lateral flexion to the left/right/reduction *frontal*
   b. also abduction/adduction
4. horizontal, transverse, or spinal rotation (left/right) *transverse*
5. circumduction *oblique/diagonal*

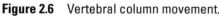

Figure 2.6   Vertebral column movement.

Scapula

1. upward rotation/downward rotation *frontal*
2. a. protraction/retraction *transverse*
   b. also adduction/abduction
3. elevation/depression *sagittal*
4. upward tilt/downward tilt *sagittal*
5. lateral tilt/medial tilt

up/down forward/back

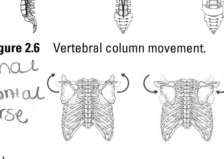

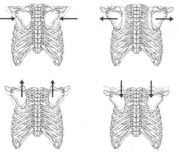

Figure 2.7   Scapular movements.

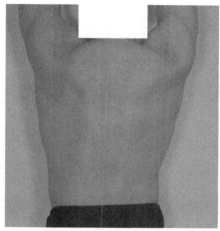

Figure 2.8   Scapula upward rotation.

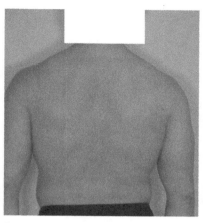

Figure 2.9   Scapula downward rotation.

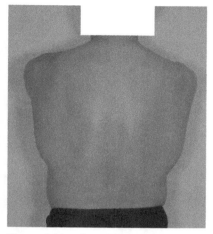

Figure 2.10   Scapula abduction (protraction).

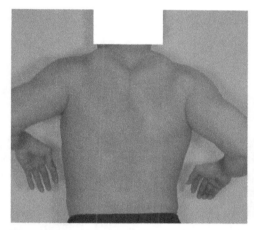

Figure 2.11   Scapula adduction (retraction).

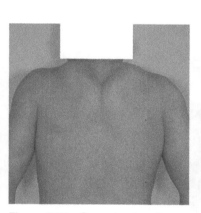

Figure 2.12   Scapula elevation.

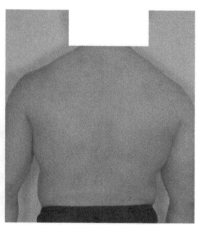

Figure 2.13   Scapula depression.

Shoulder and Hip

1. flexion/extension *sagittal*
2. hyperflexion/hyperextension
3. adduction/abduction *frontal*
4. hyperadduction/hyperabduction
5. a. medial rotation/lateral rotation
   b. also inward rotation/outward rotation *transverse*
   c. also internal rotation/external rotation
6. a. horizontal flexion/horizontal extension (cannot be performed from anatomical position)
   b. also horizontal adduction/ horizontal abduction *transverse*
   c. also transverse flexion/transverse extension
   d. also transverse adduction/ transverse abduction
7. circumduction *diagonal / oblique*
8. diagonal abduction/diagonal adduction

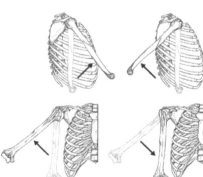

Figure 2.14   Shoulder movements.

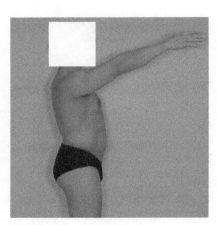

Figure 2.15   Shoulder flexion.

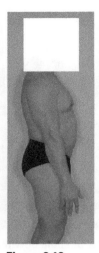

Figure 2.16
Shoulder extension.

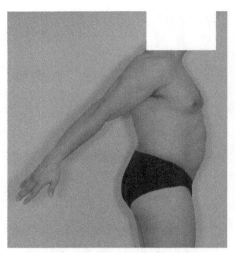

Figure 2.17   Shoulder hyperextension.

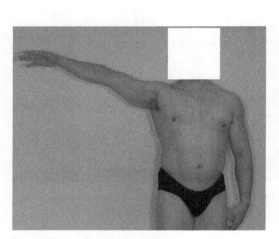

Figure 2.18   Shoulder abduction.

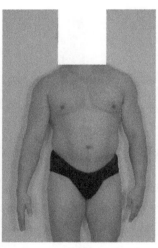

Figure 2.19   Shoulder
adduction.

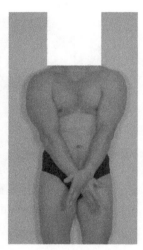

Figure 2.20   Shoulder
hyperadduction.

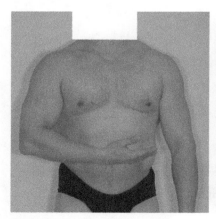

Figure 2.21   Shoulder medial
(internal, inward) rotation.

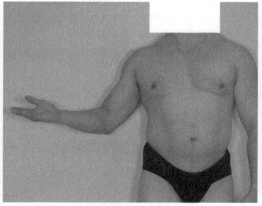

Figure 2.22   Shoulder lateral (external,
outward) rotation.

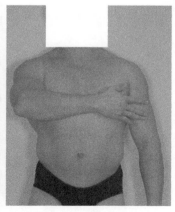

Figure 2.23   Shoulder
horizontal flexion.

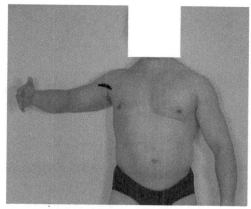

Figure 2.24 Shoulder horizontal extension.

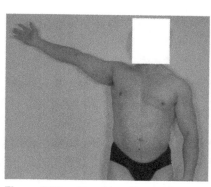

Figure 2.25 Shoulder diagonal abduction.

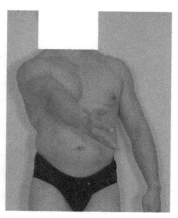

Figure 2.26 Shoulder diagonal adduction.

Note: Shoulder joint actions are accompanied by actions of the shoulder girdle (scapula).

Shoulder joint action	Shoulder girdle (scapula) action
flexion	elevation
extension	depression, downward rotation
abduction	upward rotation
adduction	downward rotation
hyperextension	upward tilt
horizontal flexion	protraction, lateral tilt
horizontal extension	retraction, medial tilt
medial rotation	protraction
lateral rotation	retraction
diagonal abduction	retraction, elevation, upward rotation
diagonal adduction	protraction, depression, downward rotation

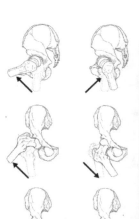

Figure 2.27 Hip joint movements.

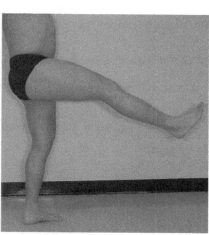

Figure 2.28 Hip flexion.

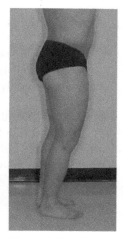

Figure 2.29 Hip extension.

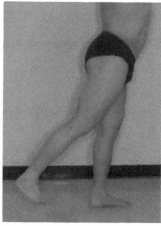

Figure 2.30 Hip hyperextension.

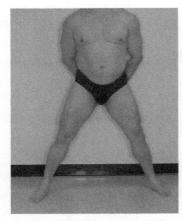

Figure 2.31   Hip abduction.

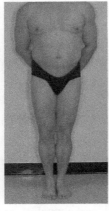

Figure 2.32   Hip adduction.

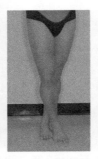

Figure 2.33   Hip hyper-adduction.

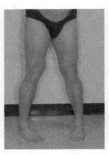

Figure 2.34   Hip medial (inward, internal) rotation.

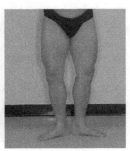

Figure 2.35   Hip lateral (outward, external) rotation.

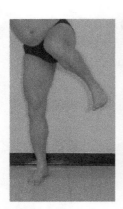

Figure 2.36   Hip horizontal flexion.

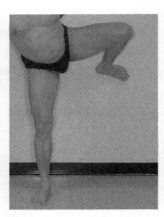

Figure 2.37   Hip horizontal extension.

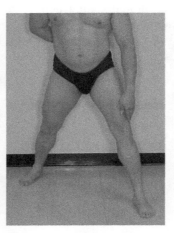

Figure 2.38   Hip diagonal abduction.

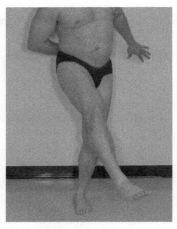

Figure 2.39   Hip diagonal adduction.

Hip only
1. a. anterior pelvic tilt/posterior pelvic tilt
   b. also anterior pelvic rotation/ posterior pelvic rotation
2. a. left lateral pelvic tilt/right lateral pelvic tilt
   b. also left lateral pelvic rotation/ right lateral pelvic rotation
3. left transverse pelvic rotation/ right transverse pelvic rotation

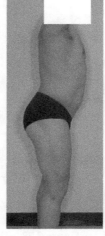

Figure 2.40   Hip anterior pelvic tilt.

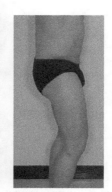

Figure 2.41   Hip posterior pelvic tilt.

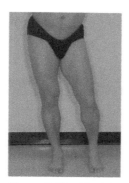

Figure 2.42 Hip left lateral pelvic tilt.

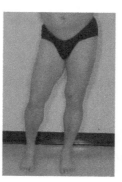

Figure 2.43 Hip right lateral pelvic tilt.

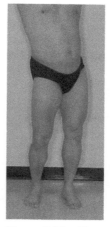

Figure 2.44 Hip left transverse pelvic rotation.

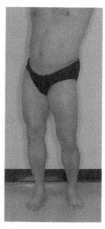

Figure 2.45 Hip right transverse pelvic rotation.

Elbow and Knee
1. flexion/extension *sagittal*
2. hyperextension

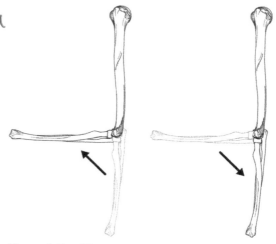

Figure 2.46   Elbow movements.

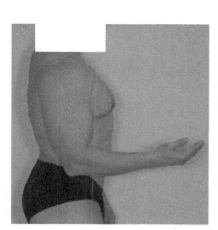

Figure 2.47   Elbow flexion.

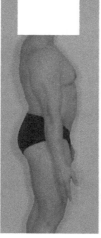

Figure 2.48 Elbow extension.

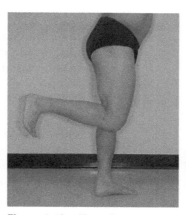

Figure 2.49   Knee flexion.

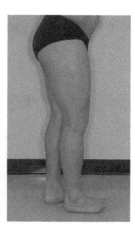

Figure 2.50   Knee extension.

Knee only
1. some medial
    rotation/lateral rotation
    when knee is flexed

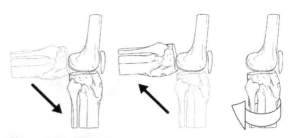

Figure 2.51   Knee movements.

Radio-Ulnar Joint (Forearm)
1. pronation/supination

transverse   *holding soup*

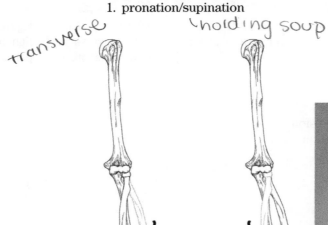

Figure 2.52   Pronation and supination.

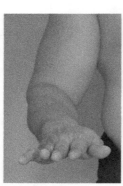

Figure 2.53   Forearm pronation.

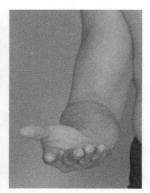

Figure 2.54   Forearm supination.

Wrist (Radio-Carpal)
1. a. flexion/extension   *sagittal*
    b. also palmar flexion/dorsal flexion
2. hyperextension
3. a. abduction/adduction   *frontal*
    b. also radial flexion/ulnar flexion
    c. also radial deviation/ulnar deviation
4. circumduction

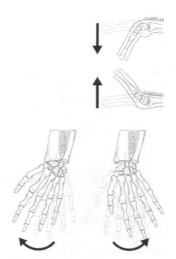

Figure 2.55   Wrist movements.

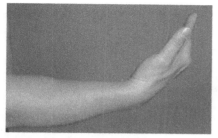

Figure 2.56   Wrist flexion.

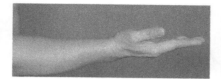

Figure 2.57   Wrist extension.

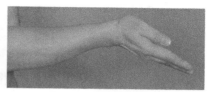

Figure 2.58   Wrist hyperextension.

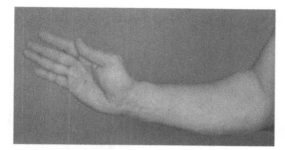

Figure 2.59   Wrist abduction (radial flexion).

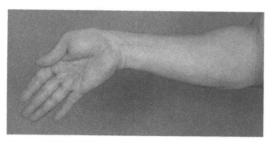

Figure 2.60   Wrist adduction (ulnar flexion).

Ankle and Foot
1. a. plantar flexion/dorsiflexion
   b. also extension/flexion
2. abduction/adduction
3. inversion/eversion
4. circumduction
5. pronation (abduction and eversion and dorsiflexion)/supination (adduction and inversion and plantar flexion)

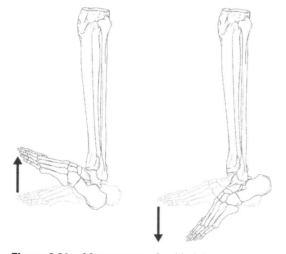

Figure 2.61   Movements of ankle joint.

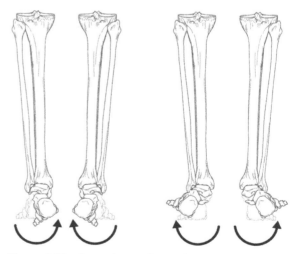

Figure 2.62   Inversion and eversion.

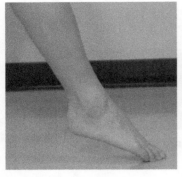

Figure 2.63 Plantar flexion (extension).

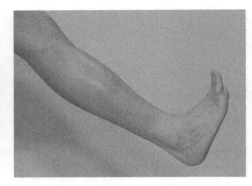

Figure 2.64 Dorsiflexion (flexion).

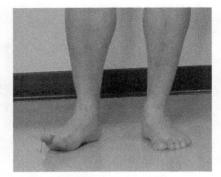

Figure 2.65 Abduction.

transverse

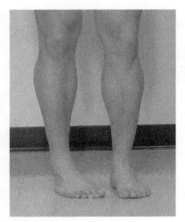

Figure 2.66 Adduction.

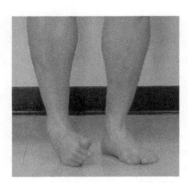

Figure 2.67 Ankle inversion.

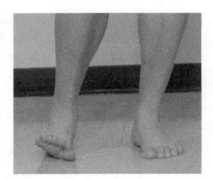

Figure 2.68 Ankle eversion.

frontal

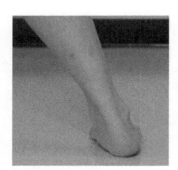

Figure 2.69 Foot pronation.

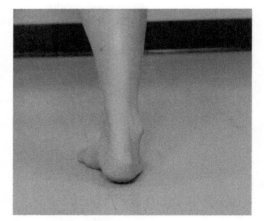

Figure 2.70 Foot supination.

Metacarpal-Phalangeal (Metatarsal-Phalangeal) Joint
1. flexion/extension
2. adduction/abduction
3. hyperextension (at the metatarsal-phalangeal joint during plantar flexion)
4. circumduction

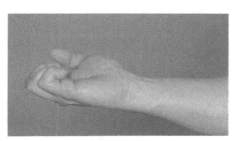

Figure 2.71   Finger flexion.

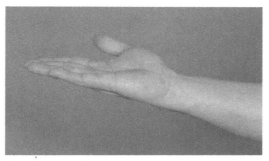

Figure 2.72   Finger extension.

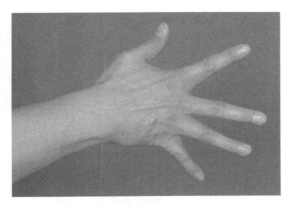

Figure 2.73   Finger abduction.

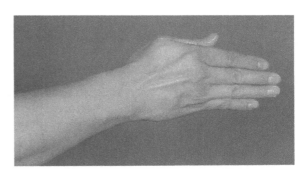

Figure 2.74   Finger adduction.

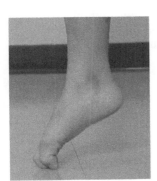

Figure 2.75   Toes flexion.

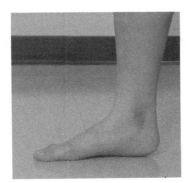

Figure 2.76   Toes extension.

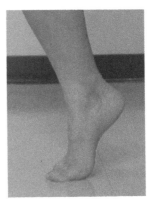

Figure 2.77   Toes hyperextension.

Inter-Phalangeal Joint
1. flexion/extension

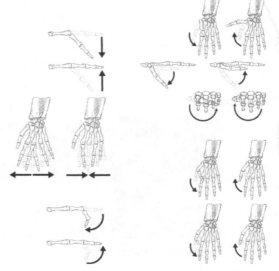

Figure 2.78   Finger
movements.

Figure 2.79   Thumb
movements.

Movement Analysis Progression

1. Learn anatomical and movement terminology
2. Develop a reference frame (planes and axes)
3. Provide examples of movement activities that occur in different planes and axes
4. Identify and demonstrate joint actions from anatomical position
5. Demonstrate all possible joint actions in different planes and axes
6. Follow movement instructions given in scientific terminology and identify the plane and axis of different joint movements
7. Provide movement instructions in scientific terminology with corresponding planes and axes to perform a skill or activity
8. Learn to break a movement activity into various phases and sub-phases
9. Identify the joint actions, planes, axes, type of contraction, and muscles involved in different phases and sub-phases of a given movement activity

↳ change from one
   position to another

Movement Instruction II

Give movement instructions in scientific terminology for the sequence of events involved in:

1. shaking hands

2. drinking a glass of water

3. throwing a baseball

4. catching a medicine ball

5. a golf swing

6. a baseball swing

7. a basketball free throw

8. a tennis forehand

9. a tennis backhand

10. shot putting

11. lifting a large box

WORKSHEET 2.6

Movement Analysis

For the following movement activities, break the skill into phases and sub-phases. Then, for each phase or sub-phase, identify:

1. the joints involved
2. the simultaneous/sequential nature of the joints involved
3. the joint types
4. the degrees of freedom of each joint
5. the starting position for each joint
6. the actions at each joint
7. the segment being moved at each joint
8. the plane and axis the movement is occurring in

1. Standing Toe Touch

Simultaneous or Sequential?

Phases	Joints	Joint Type	Degrees of Freedom	Starting Position	Observed Joint Action	Segment Moved	Plane	Axis

2. Squat

Simultaneous or Sequential?

Phases	Joints	Joint Type	Degrees of Freedom	Starting Position	Observed Joint Action	Segment Moved	Plane	Axis

Phases	Joints	Joint Type	Degrees of Freedom	Starting Position	Observed Joint Action	Segment Moved	Plane	Axis

3. Sit-Up

Simultaneous or Sequential?

Phases	Joints	Joint Type	Degrees of Freedom	Starting Position	Observed Joint Action	Segment Moved	Plane	Axis

Phases	Joints	Joint Type	Degrees of Freedom	Starting Position	Observed Joint Action	Segment Moved	Plane	Axis

4. Overhead Press

Simultaneous or Sequential?

Phases	Joints	Joint Type	Degrees of Freedom	Starting Position	Observed Joint Action	Segment Moved	Plane	Axis

Phases	Joints	Joint Type	Degrees of Freedom	Starting Position	Observed Joint Action	Segment Moved	Plane	Axis

5. Pull Up

Simultaneous or Sequential?

Phases	Joints	Joint Type	Degrees of Freedom	Starting Position	Observed Joint Action	Segment Moved	Plane	Axis

Phases	Joints	Joint Type	Degrees of Freedom	Starting Position	Observed Joint Action	Segment Moved	Plane	Axis

6. Push Up

Simultaneous or Sequential?

Phases	Joints	Joint Type	Degrees of Freedom	Starting Position	Observed Joint Action	Segment Moved	Plane	Axis

Phases	Joints	Joint Type	Degrees of Freedom	Starting Position	Observed Joint Action	Segment Moved	Plane	Axis

PART II

Muscles of the Axial and Appendicular Skeleton

Fixators, stabilizers -

   muscles that contract statically
(isometrically) to steady or support
 some part of the body against the
 pull of gravity, or against any
 other force that interferes w/ the
 desired movement (e.g. back
    extensor involvement) in the performance
 of arm curls

Neutralizers - muscles which act to prevent
    an undesired action of agonists
  (e.g. biceps brachii causes supination
   of the forearm + flexion of elbow joint.
   If only flexion of elbow is desired from
  the fundamental position w/o supination,
   the pronator teres would contract to
   neutralize the supination actions)

CHAPTER 3

Muscles of the Trunk and Neck

Objectives

To be able to:
1. determine how muscles are named and the roles of muscle
2. locate and identify the muscles that act on the trunk and neck
3. identify the actions of a given muscle at the trunk and neck
4. identify the muscles of the trunk involved in a given action or activity
5. identify and locate the origins and insertions of the muscles of the trunk

Muscle Terminology

Origin—Classical Definition—The proximal attachment site of a muscle.

—Functional Definition—The attachment site of a muscle on the stable (non-moving) segment of a single-joint system.

Insertion—Classical Definition—The distal attachment site of a muscle.

—Functional Definition—The attachment site of a muscle on the moving segment of a single-joint system.

Action—The function of a muscle as defined when the muscle shortens as it contracts.

A muscle has two parts:
1. belly
2. tendons—connect muscle to bone

Note: Since a muscle can *only* try to pull its two ends together, the action of a muscle is defined as if the muscle is "doing what it wants to do." When the muscle shortens as it contracts, the distance between the origin and insertion points decreases.

Agonist—The prime mover: a muscle primarily associated with a given action. *Important in de accerelation*

Synergist—A muscle that assists the agonist.

Antagonist—A muscle whose action is opposite that of the agonist.

Stabilizer/Fixator—A muscle whose action is recruited to eliminate undesired bony actions.

Neutralizer—A muscle whose action is recruited to eliminate undesired muscle actions.

Muscles are named according to:
1. function
2. heads (number of heads)
3. size
4. location
5. attachments
6. shape

Function

1. abduction—*abductor* pollicis longus
2. adduction—*adductor* magnus
3. flexion—*flexor* carpi radialis
4. extension—*extensor* digiti minimi
5. elevation—*levator* scapulae
6. pronation—*pronator* teres
7. supination—*supinator*
8. plantar flexion—*plantaris* longus

Number of Heads

1. two—*bi*ceps femoris
2. three—*tri*ceps brachii
3. four—*quad*riceps femoris

Size

1. big—psoas *major*, adductor *magnus*
2. small—pectoralis *minor*
3. short—peroneus *brevis*
4. long—adductor *longus*

Location

1. above—*supra*spinatus
2. below—*infra*spinatus
3. front—*anterior* deltoid
4. back—*posterior* deltoid
5. deep—*internal* oblique
6. superficial—*external* oblique
7. brachial—*brachialis*, biceps *brachii*
8. pectoral—*pectoralis* major
9. gluteal—*gluteus* maximus
10. palm—*palmaris* longus
11. abdominal—rectus *abdominis*
12. femoral—rectus *femoris*
13. medial—vastus *medialis*
14. lateral—vastus *lateralis*
15. between—vastus *intermedius*

Attachments

1. sternocleidomastoid
2. subclavius
3. coracobrachialis
4. brachioradialis
5. flexor carpi ulnaris
6. tibialis anterior
7. quadratus lumborum
8. erector spinae
9. levator scapulae

Shape

1. round—*teres* major
2. triangle—anterior *deltoid*
3. square—pronator *quadratus*

4. sawtooth—*serratus* anterior
5. kite shaped—*rhomboid* major
6. trapezoid—*trapezius*
7. running diagonally—internal *oblique*
8. widest or broadest—*latissimus* dorsi

Muscles of the Trunk and Neck

Rectus Abdominis

Origin—anterior surface of pubic crest
Insertion—xiphoid process, anterior cartilage of 5th, 6th and 7th ribs
Actions—Trunk—flexion when both sides contract
       —lateral flexion when one side contracts
     —decreases curvature of lumbar region of vertebral column

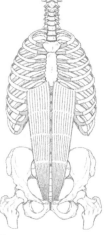

Figure 3.1 Rectus abdominis muscle.

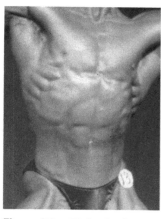

Figure 3.2 Abdominals (relaxed).

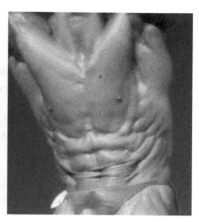

Figure 3.3 Abdominals (contracted).

External Oblique (Obliquus Externus Abdominus)

Origin—inferior border of lower 8 ribs (ribs 5–12)
Insertion—anterior one-half of iliac crest, pubic crest, linea alba
Actions—Trunk—flexion when both sides contract
       —lateral flexion to the same side and rotation to opposite side when one side contracts

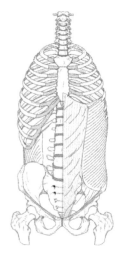

Figure 3.4 External oblique muscle.

Internal Oblique (Obliquus Internus Abdominus)

Origin—lateral upper one-half of inguinal ligament,
        anterior one-half to two-thirds of iliac crest,
        lumbar fascia

Insertion—costal cartilage of ribs 7–10, linea alba

Actions—Trunk—flexion when both sides contract
        —lateral flexion to the same side and
        rotation to same side when one side
        contracts

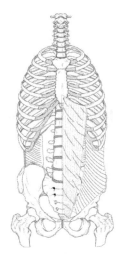

Figure 3.5 Internal oblique muscle.

Transversus Abdominus

Origin—lateral one-third of inguinal ligament, anterior two-thirds of iliac
        crest, inner surface of cartilage of lower 6 ribs, lumbar fascia

Insertion—iliopectineal line, pubic crest, linea alba

Actions—compression of abdomen (pulls abdominal wall in)
        —strong muscle of exhalation
        —stabilizes trunk

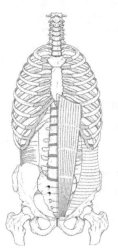

Figure 3.6
Transversus
abdominis muscle.

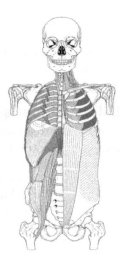

Figure 3.7 Body
wall muscles.

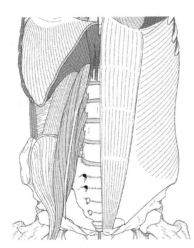

Figure 3.8 Abdominal body wall
muscles.

Quadratus Lumborum

Origin—posterior iliac crest and iliolumbar ligament
Insertion—lower border of 12th rib, transverse
          processes of first 4 lumbar vertebrae (L1–L4)
Actions—Trunk—lateral flexion when one side con-
          tracts
          —stabilization of pelvis and lumbar
          spine when both sides contract
          —extension

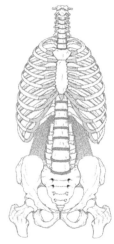

Figure 3.9
Quadratus
lumborum muscle.

Deep Posterior Spinal Muscles

1. Multifidi
2. Rotatores
3. Levatores Costarum
4. Interspinales
5. Intertransversarii

Origin—posterior portions of all
        vertebrae, posterior surface
        of sacrum
Insertion—spinous and transverse
        processes and laminae
        just above those on
        which the muscle portion
        originates
Actions—extends and hyperextends
        spine (when both sides
        contract)
        —rotation of spine to oppo-
        site side, lateral flexion
        (when one side contracts)

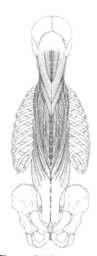

Figure 3.10
Vertebral extensor
muscles.

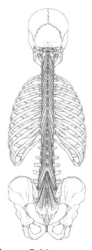

Figure 3.11
Multifidus muscle.

Erector Spinae (Sacrospinalis)

1. Iliocostalis (lumborum, thoracis, cervicis)
2. Longissimus (thoracis, cervicis, capitis)
3. Spinalis (thoracis, cervicis, capitis)

Origin—ligamentum nuchae, spinous and transverse processes of lumbar,
        thoracic and cervical vertebrae, lower nine ribs, posterior surface of
        sacrum, and posterior iliac crest
Insertion—each fiber passes in a superior or a superior and lateral direction
        to the spinous, transverse processes of the lumbar, thoracic, cervi-
        cal vertebrae, angles of the 12 ribs, and mastoid process of tempo-
        ral bone.

Actions—extension and hyperextension of head and spine when all branches
are contracting

—lateral flexion when one side contracts in conjunction with lateral
and anterior muscles of the same side

—rotation of the head and spine to same side of the contracting
muscle (when combined with contraction of various lateral and
anterior muscles)

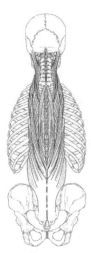

Figure 3.12   Erector spinae muscles.

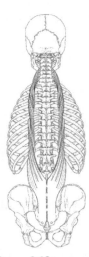

Figure 3.13
Iliocostis muscle.

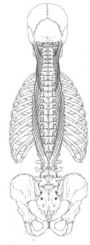

Figure 3.14
Longissimus muscle.

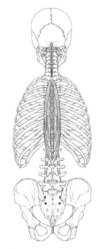

Figure 3.15
Spinalis muscle.

Semispinalis (Thoracic, Cervicis, Capitis)

Origin—transverse processes of all thoracic and 7th
cervical vertebrae, articular processes of lower
4 cervical vertebrae

Insertion—spinous process of upper 4 thoracic and
lower 5 cervical vertebrae; occipital

Actions—extension and hyperextension of thoracic and
cervical spine (when both sides contract)

—lateral flexion, rotation to the opposite side
(when one side contracts)

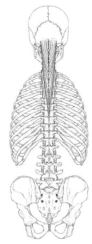

Figure 3.16
Semispinalis muscle.

Sternocleidomastoid

Origin—manubrium of sternum and
   third of clavicle
Insertion—mastoid process of temporal
   bone
Actions—flexion of head and neck
   (when both sides contract)
   —lateral flexion of neck to the
   same side and rotation to the
   opposite side (when one side
   contracts)

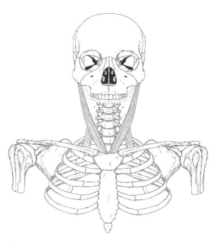

Figure 3.17
Sternocleidomastoid muscle.

Scalenus (Anterior, Medius, Posterior)

Origin—upper two ribs
Insertion—transverse processes of vertebrae C2–C6
Actions—flexion of head and neck (when both sides contract)
   —lateral flexion (when one side contracts)

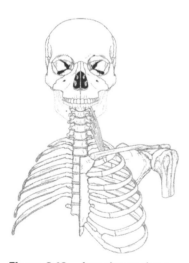

Figure 3.18   Anterior scalene
muscle.

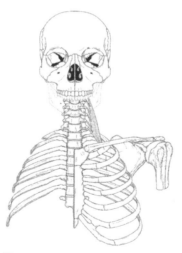

Figure 3.19   Middle scalene
muscle.

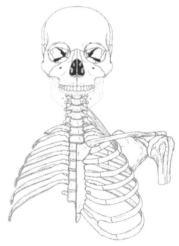

Figure 3.20   Posterior scalene
muscle.

Splenius (Capitis, Cervicis)

Origin—lower half of ligamentum nuchae, spinous processes of vertebrae T12–C6

Insertion—mastoid process of temporal bone, transverse processes of vertebrae C1–C3.

Actions—extension and hyperextension of head and neck (when both sides contract)

—lateral flexion and rotation to the same side (when one side contracts)

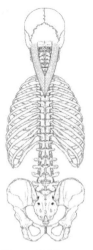

Figure 3.21
Splenius capitis muscle.

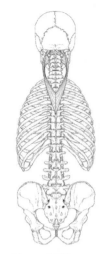

Figure 3.22
Splenius cervicis muscle.

Summary of Actions at the Trunk and Neck

Flexion

1. Rectus Abdominis
2. Obliquus Externus Abdominis
3. Obliquus Internus Abdominis
4. Sternocleidomastoid
5. Scalenus (anterior, medius, posterior)

Extension and Hyperextension

1. Erector Spinae (longissimus, spinalis, iliocostalis)
2. Deep Posterior Spinal Muscles (multifidi, rotatores, interspinales, intertransversarii, levatores costarum)
3. Semispinalis (thoracic, cervicis, capitis)
4. Splenius (capitis, cervicis)

Lateral Flexion (When One Side Contracts)

1. Rectus Abdominis
2. Obliquus Externus Abdominis
3. Obliquus Internus Abdominis
4. Quadratus Lumborum
5. Deep Posterior Spinal Muscles
6. Erector Spinae
7. Semispinalis
8. Sternocleidomastoid
9. Scalenus (anterior, medius, posterior)
10. Splenius (capitis, cervicis)

Rotation to the Same Side

1. Obliquus Internus Abdominis
2. Erector Spinae
3. Splenius (capitis, cervicis)

Rotation to the Opposite Side

1. Obliquus Externus Abdominis
2. Deep Posterior Spinal Muscles
3. Semispinalis
4. Sternocleidomastoid

Table 3.1. Trunk Muscle Action Chart

	Rect. Ab.		Ext. Obl.		Int. Obl.		Quad. L.		Erector		D. Post.	
Action	R	L	R	L	R	L	R	L	R	L	R	L
Flexion	✓	✓	✓	✓	✓	✓						
Extension									✓	✓	✓	✓
Lat. Flex R	✓		✓		✓		✓		✓		✓	
Lat. Flex L		✓		✓		✓		✓		✓		✓
Rotation R				✓	✓				✓			✓
Rotation L			✓			✓				✓	✓	

Table 3.2. Neck Muscle Action Chart

	Sterno.		Scalenes		Splenius		Subocc.		Erector		D. Post.	
Action	R	L	R	L	R	L	R	L	R	L	R	L
Flexion	✓	✓	✓	✓								
Extension					✓	✓	✓	✓	✓	✓	✓	✓
Lat. Flex R	✓		✓		✓				✓		✓	
Lat. Flex L		✓		✓		✓				✓		✓
Rotation R		✓			✓		✓		✓			✓
Rotation L	✓					✓		✓		✓	✓	

WORKSHEET 3.1

Muscles of the Trunk and Neck

Muscles	Origin	Insertion	Actions
Rectus Abdominis	_____	_____	flex, lat flex, decr. lumbar curve
External Oblique	_____	_____	flex, lat flex, opp rot
Internal Oblique	_____	_____	flex, lat flex, same rot
Transverse Abdominis	_____	_____	compression, stabilization
Quadratus Lumborum	_____	_____	lat flex, stabilization
Deep Posterior Spinal Muscles			
Multifidi	_____	_____	ext, hyperext, lat flex, opp rot
Rotatores	_____	_____	ext, hyperext, lat flex, opp rot
Levatores Costarum	_____	_____	ext, hyperext, lat flex, opp rot
Interspinales	_____	_____	ext, hyperext, lat flex, opp rot
Erector Spinae (Sacrospinalis)			
Longissimus	_____	_____	ext, hyperext, lat flex, same rot
Spinalis	_____	_____	ext, hyperext, lat flex, same rot
Iliocostalis	_____	_____	ext, hyperext, lat flex, same rot
Semispinalis			
Thoracic	_____	_____	ext, hyperext, lat flex, opp rot
Cervicis	_____	_____	ext, hyperext, lat flex, opp rot
Capitis	_____	_____	ext, hyperext, lat flex, opp rot
Sternocleidomastoid	_____	_____	flex, lat flex, opp rot
Scalenus			
Anterior	_____	_____	flex, lat flex
Medius	_____	_____	flex, lat flex
Posterior	_____	_____	flex, lat flex
Splenius			
Capitis	_____	_____	ext, hyperext, lat flex, same rot
Cervicis	_____	_____	ext, hyperext, lat flex, same rot

Muscles of the Trunk and Neck

For the following pictures, identify (with arrows) as many muscles as possible.

1.

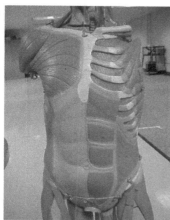

2.

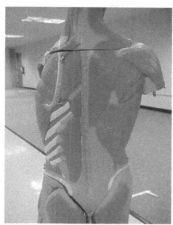

3.

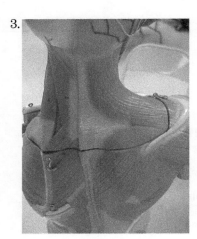

WORKSHEET 3.3

Muscles of the Trunk and Neck

1. Flexion of the Neck and Head
   Subject: Lie on the back and lift the head by bringing the chin toward the chest.
   1) Palpate the sternocleidomastoid.
   2) Perform the same movement from a standing position. What is the motive force, what muscle is contracting, and what type of contraction is performed?
2. Extension (Hyperextension) of the Neck and Head
   Subject: Lie face down on a table with the head over the edge. Raise the head as far as possible.
   Assistant: May resist the movement if necessary.
   1) Palpate and identify as many contracting muscles as possible. What muscles do you expect to contract?
   2) Perform the same movement from a standing position. What is the motive force, what muscle is contracting, and what type of contraction is performed? Does this change during the range of motion of the movement?
3. Lateral Flexion of the Neck and Head
   Subject: Lie on one side and raise the head toward the shoulder without turning the head or tensing the shoulder.
   Assistant: Give slight resistance to the side of the head.
   1) Palpate and identify as many contracting muscles as possible. What muscles do you expect to contract?
4. Rotation of the Neck and Head
   Subject: In a sitting position, rotate the head to the left as far as possible.
   Assistant: Give fairly strong resistant to the jaw.
   1) Palpate the sternocleidomastoids. Which side contracts?
5. Flexion of the Thoracic and Lumbar Spine
   Subject: Lie on the back with arms folded across the chest. Flex the head, shoulders, and upper back from the table, keeping the chin near the chest. Do not flex the hips.
   Assistant: Hold the thighs down.
   1) Palpate the rectus abdominus and external obliques.
6. Extension (Hyperextension) of the Thoracic and Lumbar Spine
   Subject: Lie face down with the hands on the hips. Hyperextend the head and trunk as far as possible.
   Assistant: Hold the feet down.
   1) Palpate the erector spinae.
   2) Palpate the gluteus maximus. Is this muscle contracting? If so, what is its function?
7. Lateral Flexion of the Thoracic and Lumbar Spine
   Subject: Lie on one side with the inferior arm across the chest, its hand on the opposite shoulder, and the superior arm resting on the hip. Laterally flex the trunk.
   Assistant: Hold the legs down. If necessary, help the subject by pulling at the elbow.
   1) Palpate the rectus abdominus, external oblique, and erector spinae.
   2) Is the latissimus dorsi active? Why or why not? Does it matter if the assistant is pulling on the elbow?

8. Rotation of the Thoracic and Lumbar Spine

   Subject: Sit on a chair with the hands placed behind the neck and rotate to one side as far as possible without leaving the chair.

   Assistant: Resist the movement by grasping the subject's arms close to the shoulders and resisting the movement.

   1) Palpate and identify as many of the contracting muscles as possible. Disregard the muscles of the scapula and the arm.

9. Flexion of Lumbar Region of Vertebral Column

   Subject: Lying supine on back, flex hips by doing a leg raise with both legs.

   Assistant: Resist the movement by applying force downwards on the subject's ankles.

   1) What happens to the lumbar region of the vertebral column during hip flexion?

   2) How can you decrease flexion of the lumbar region of the vertebral column?

CHAPTER 4

Muscles of the Shoulder Girdle (Scapula)

Objectives

To be able to:
1. locate and identify the muscles that act on the shoulder girdle
2. identify the actions of a given muscle at the shoulder girdle
3. identify the muscles of the shoulder girdle involved in a given action or activity
4. identify and locate the origins and insertions of the muscles of the shoulder girdle
5. identify the muscles of the shoulder girdle when given the origins and/or insertions
6. determine from the origins and insertions, the muscles action(s) on the shoulder girdle
7. determine the muscles recruited for isolated movements of the scapula

Muscles of the Shoulder Girdle (Sternum/Clavicle/Scapula)

Trapezius

Origin—(Part 1)—occipital protuberance at base of skull
  —(Part 2)—ligamentum nuchae (ligaments of neck)
  —(Part 3)—spinous process of vertebrae C7 and T1–T3
  —(Part 4)—spinous process of vertebrae T4–T12

Insertion—(Part 1)—posterior lateral one-third of clavicle
  —(Part 2)—acromion process
  —(Part 3)—superior border of scapular spine
  —(Part 4)—proximal end (root) of scapular spine

Actions—(Part 1)—elevation (if origins and insertions reversed, transverse rotation of the head to the opposite side if one side contracts, extension and hyperextension of the head if both sides contract)
  —(Part 2)—elevation, upward rotation, adduction, medial tilt
  —(Part 3)—adduction, medial tilt
  —(Part 4)—depression, upward rotation, adduction, medial tilt

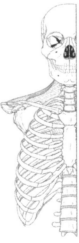

Figure 4.1 Trapezius muscle, anterior view.

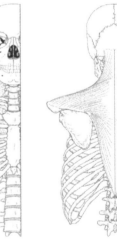

Figure 4.2 Trapezius muscle, posterior view.

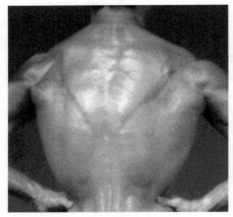

Figure 4.3   Trapezius (relaxed).

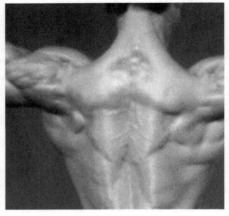

Figure 4.4   Trapezius (contracted).

Levator Scapulae

Origin—transverse processes of vertebrae C1–C4

Insertion—medial border of scapula above scapular spine

Actions—elevation, downward rotation (lateral flexion of head when only one side contracts and when the origins and insertions are reversed)

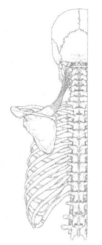

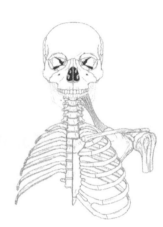

Figure 4.5   Levator scapulae muscle.

Figure 4.6   Levator scapulae.

Rhomboids Major and Minor

Origin—(Minor)—spinous process of vertebrae C7–T1

—(Major)—spinous process of vertebrae T2–T5

Insertion—(Minor)—medial border of scapula at the scapular spine

—(Major)—medial border of scapula between the spine and inferior angle

Actions—elevation, adduction, downward rotation, medial tilt

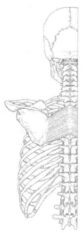

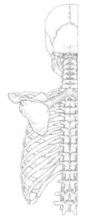

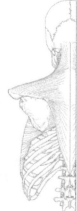

Figure 4.7 Rhomboideus major muscle.

Figure 4.8 Rhomboideus minor muscle.

Figure 4.9 Scapular muscles, posterior view.

Pectoralis Minor

Origin—superior anterior surface of 3rd, 4th, and 5th ribs
Insertion—coracoid process of scapula
Actions—abduction, lateral tilt, downward rotation, up-
ward tilt, depression

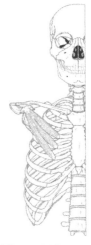

Figure 4.10
Pectoralis minor
muscle.

Serratus Anterior

Origin—lateral surface of ribs 1–9
Insertion—anterior medial border of scapula
Actions—abduction, upward rotation, lateral tilt

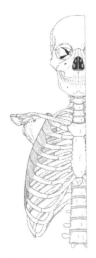

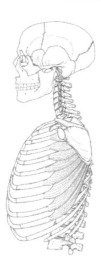

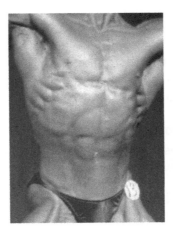

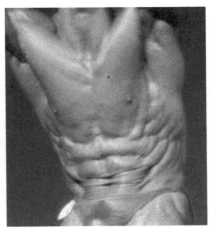

Figure 4.11
Serratus anterior
muscle, anterior
view.

Figure 4.12
Serratus anterior
muscle, lateral
view.

Figure 4.13   Serratus anterior
(trunk extended).

Figure 4.14   Serratus anterior (trunk
flexed).

Subclavius

Origin—superior surface of 1st rib and costal cartilage

Insertion—inferior surface of middle one-third of clavicle

Actions—protects and stabilizes sternoclavicular joint (assists in abduction, downward rotation, depression)

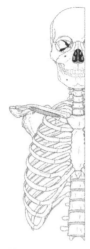

Figure 4.15
Subclavius
muscle.

Summary of Actions at the Shoulder Girdle

Abduction (Protraction)

1. Serratus Anterior
2. Pectoralis Minor
3. Assistant (subclavius)

Adduction (Retraction)

1. Rhomboids Major and Minor
2. Trapezius (Part 2, 3, 4)

Upward Rotation

1. Serratus Anterior
2. Trapezius (Part 2, 4)

Downward Rotation

1. Rhomboids Major and Minor
2. Pectoralis Minor
3. Levator Scapulae
4. Assistant (subclavius)

Elevation

1. Levator Scapulae
2. Rhomboids Major and Minor
3. Trapezius (Part 1, 2)

Depression

1. Pectoralis Minor
2. Trapezius (Part 4)
3. Assistant (subclavius)

Lateral Tilt

1. Serratus Anterior
2. Pectoralis Minor

Medial Tilt

1. Trapezius (Part 2, 3, 4)
2. Rhomboids Major and Minor

Upward Tilt

1. Pectoralis Minor

Table 4.1. Shoulder Girdle Muscle Action Chart

Action	Pec. Min.	Trap I	Trap II	Trap III	Trap IV	Rhomb.	S. Ant.	L. Scap.
Elev.		✓	✓			✓		✓
Dep.	✓				✓			
Ab./Pro.	✓						✓	
Ad./Ret.			✓	✓	✓	✓		
Up Rot.			✓		✓		✓	
D. Rot.	✓						✓	✓
Lat Tilt	✓						✓	
Med Tilt			✓	✓	✓	✓		
Up Tilt	✓							

also:
lat. flex.
of cerv.
spine

WORKSHEET 4.1

Muscles of the Shoulder Girdle

Muscles	Origin	Insertion	Actions
Trapezius			
Part 1	_____	_____	elev.
Part 2	_____	_____	elev., upward rot, add, med. tilt
Part 3	_____	_____	add, med tilt
Part 4	_____	_____	depr. upward rot, add, med tilt
Serratus Anterior	_____	_____	abd, upward rot, lat tilt
Pectoralis Minor	_____	_____	abd, downward rot, depression, upward tilt, lateral tilt
Levator Scapulae	_____	_____	elevation, downward rot
Rhomboids	_____	_____	elev, downward rot, adduction, med tilt
Subclavius	_____	_____	stabilizes sternoclavicular joint

Muscles of the Shoulder Girdle

The Determination of Muscle Recruitment for Isolated Movements

Determine the muscles recruited for the following movements at the scapula (based on the method used for the example below).

1. Adduction (retraction)
2. Upward Rotation
3. Downward Rotation
4. Depression

Example

1. Pick a joint and a specific action (e.g., scapula elevation).

Scapula—Elevation			

2. List ALL muscles that produce the specific action selected (e.g., trapezius, part I and II; rhomboids; levator scapulae).

Scapula—Elevation			
Trap I	**Trap II**	**Rhomboid**	**Lev. Scap.**

3. List ALL of the actions of ALL of the muscles listed, beginning with the desired action. List the order of the actions in the same order for each listed muscle.

	Scapula—Elevation			
	Trap I	Trap II	Rhomboid	Lev. Scap.
All Actions	**Elevation**	**Elevation** **Up. Rot.** **Adduction**	**Elevation** **Down. Rot.** **Adduction**	**Elevation** **Down. Rot.**

4. Eliminate (cross off) all undesired agonist-antagonistic pairs of actions.

	Scapula—Elevation			
	Trap I	Trap II	Rhomboid	Lev. Scap.
All Actions	**Elevation**	**Elevation** ~~Up. Rot.~~ Adduction	**Elevation** ~~Down. Rot.~~ Adduction	**Elevation** ~~Down. Rot.~~

5. For any remaining undesired actions, find another muscle (not on your current list) that will act as a neutralizer or stabilizer. This muscle cannot be antagonistic to the agonists (see second example). If there are no remaining undesired actions, your chart is complete. (*Remember that the body's own mass and external objects are often used as stabilizers, which would eliminate the need for muscular recruitment in stabilization.*)

Scapula—Elevation				
	Trap I	Trap II	Rhomboid	Lev. Scap	Serr. Ant.
All Actions	Elevation	Elevation ~~Up. Rot.~~ ~~Adduction~~	Elevation ~~Down. Rot.~~ ~~Adduction~~	Elevation ~~Down. Rot.~~	~~Up. Rot.~~ ~~Abduction~~

Scapula—Abduction				
	Serr. Ant.	Pec. Minor	Rhomboid	Lev. Scap.
All Actions	**Abduction** ~~Up. Rot.~~	~~Down. Rot.~~ ~~Depression~~	~~Down. Rot.~~ ~~Elevation~~ ~~Adduction~~	~~Down. Rot.~~ ~~Elevation~~

6. Repeat steps 3, 4, and 5 until there are no remaining undesired actions.

Scapula—Adduction				
All Actions				

Scapula—Upward Rotation				
All Actions				

Scapula—Downward Rotation				
All Actions				

Scapula—Depression				
All Actions				

Name _____   Lab Section _____

Muscles of the Shoulder Girdle

Muscle Action at the Scapula

1. Adduction/Retraction of the shoulder girdle (scapula)
   Subject: Standing with shoulders flexed 90 degrees, elbows fully flexed, and fingers resting on the shoulders, horizontally extend the shoulders.
   Assistant: Stand facing subject and resist movement by pulling on elbows.
   1) Palpate the trapezius, parts II, III, and IV.
2. Abduction/Protraction of the shoulder girdle (scapula)
   Subject: Standing with arms abducted 90 degrees, elbows fully flexed, and fingers resting on the shoulders, horizontally flex the shoulders attempting to touch the elbows in front of the chest.
   Assistant: Stand behind the subject and resist the movement by pulling on the elbows.
   1) Palpate the serratus anterior.
   2) Are any other muscles active?
3. Elevation of the shoulder girdle (scapula)
   Subject: Standing, elevate the shoulder girdle keeping the arm muscles relaxed.
   Assistant: Resist movement by exerting pressure downward on the shoulder.
   1) Palpate the trapezius, parts I and II.
   2) Try the movement again forcefully. Are any other muscles active?
4. Depression of the shoulder girdle (scapula)
   Subject: Standing with the shoulder girdle elevated and elbow flexed, push down with the elbow.
   Assistant: Resist movement by exerting pressure upward on the elbow.
   1) Palpate the trapezius, part IV.
   2) Try the movement again forcefully. Are any other muscles active?
5. Abduction of the shoulder
   Scapula: upward rotation of the scapula
   Subject: Standing, abduct the shoulder to 90 degrees with elbow fully extended. DO NOT elevate the shoulder.
   Assistant: Resist movement by exerting pressure downward on subject's elbow.
   1) Palpate the four parts of the trapezius and tell which parts contract.
6. Adduction of the shoulder
   Scapula: downward rotation and probably some adduction
   Subject: Standing with arm abducted 90 degrees, adduct arm 45 degrees.
   Assistant: Resist movement by exerting pressure upward on subject's elbow.
   1) Palpate the four parts of the trapezius and tell which parts contract.

CHAPTER 5

Muscles of the Shoulder Joint

Objectives

To be able to:
1. locate and identify the muscles that act on the shoulder joint
2. identify the actions of a given muscle at the shoulder joint
3. identify the muscles of the shoulder joint involved in a given action or activity
4. identify and locate the origins and insertions of the muscles of the shoulder joint
5. group the various muscles of the shoulder joint according to common origins, insertions, and/or actions
6. identify the muscles of the shoulder joint when given the origins and/or insertions
7. determine from the origins and insertions, the muscles action(s) on the shoulder joint

Muscle of the Shoulder Joint

Pectoralis Major

Origin—(Clavicular portion)—anterior surface of medial half of clavicle
    —(Sternal portion)—anterior surface of sternum
Insertion—inferior two-thirds of lateral lip of intertubercular groove (bicipital groove) of humerus
Actions—(Clavicular portion)—flexion, horizontal flexion, medial rotation
    —(Sternal portion)—extension, horizontal flexion, medial rotation, adduction

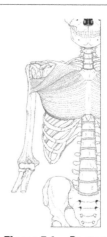

Figure 5.1 Pectoralis major muscle.

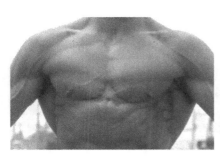

Figure 5.2 Pectoralis major (sternal and clavicular portion relaxed).

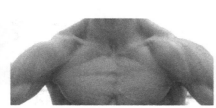

Figure 5.3 Pectoralis major (clavicular portion contracted).

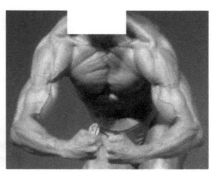

Figure 5.4 Pectoralis major (sternal and clavicular portion contracted).

103

Deltoid

Origin—(Anterior deltoid)—anterior
lateral one-third of clavicle
—(Middle deltoid)—acromion
process
—(Posterior deltoid)—scapula
spine
Insertion—deltoid tuberosity
Actions—(Anterior deltoid)—flexion,
horizontal flexion, medial
rotation
(assists in abduction)
—(Middle deltoid)—abduction
—(Posterior deltoid)—extension,
horizontal extension, lateral
rotation (assists in abduction)

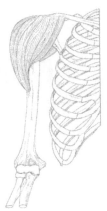

Figure 5.5
Deltoid muscle,
anterior view.

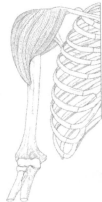

Figure 5.6
Deltoid muscle,
posterior view.

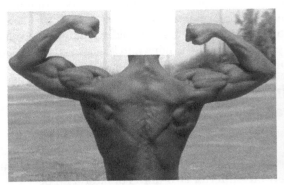

Figure 5.7   Shoulder muscles (posterior view).

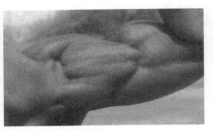

Figure 5.8   Deltoid (anterior, middle, posterior).

Coracobrachialis

Origin—coracoid process of scapula
Insertion—mid-medial shalf of humerus
Actions—flexion, horizontal flexion, adduction

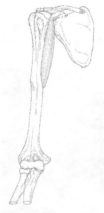

Figure 5.9
Coracobrachialis
muscle.

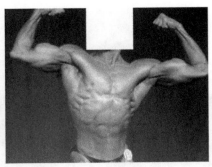

Figure 5.10   Shoulder muscle
(anterior view).

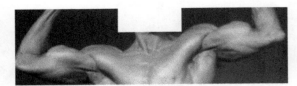

Figure 5.11   Coracobrachialis.

Latissimus Dorsi

Origin—posterior half of iliac crest; spinous processes (T6–T12, L1–L5);
   posterior surface of sacrum; lower 3 ribs
Insertion—medial side of intertubecular groove of humerus
Actions—extension, adduction, horizontal extension, medial rotation

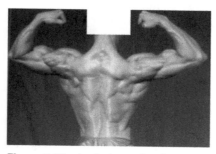

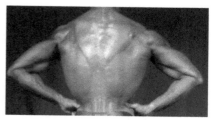

Figure 5.12 Latissimus dorsi muscle.

Figure 5.13 Latissimus dorsi (contracted).

Figure 5.14 Latissimus dorsi (relaxed).

Teres Major

Origin—lower one-third of lateral border of scapula
Insertion—inferior half of medial lip of intertubecular groove of humerus
Actions—extension, adduction, horizontal extension, medial rotation

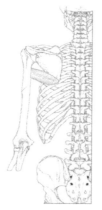

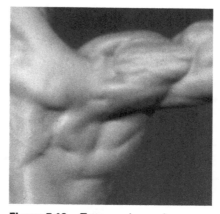

Figure 5.15 Teres major muscle.

Figure 5.16 Teres major and infraspinatus.

Teres Minor

Origin—superior two-thirds of
   posterior surface of lateral
   border of scapula
Insertion—greater tubercle of humerus
Actions—lateral rotation (also assists
   in extension, horizontal
   extension, adduction)

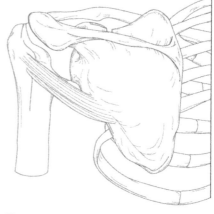

Figure 5.17 Teres minor muscle.

Infraspinatus

Origin—medial two-thirds of infra-
      spinous fossa of scapula
Insertion—greater tubercle of humerus
Actions—lateral rotation (also assists
      in extension, horizontal
      extension, adduction)

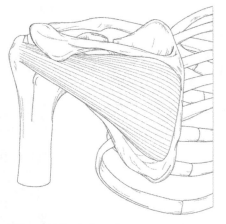

Figure 5.18   Infraspinatus muscle.

Supraspinatus

Origin—medial two-thirds of
      supraspinous fossa of scapula
Insertion—greater tubercle of humerus
Actions—abduction and stabilization of
      humerus

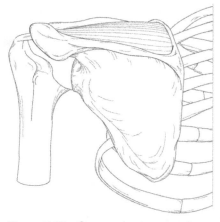

Figure 5.19   Supraspinatus muscle.

Subscapularis

Origin—subscapular fossa
Insertion—lesser tubercle of humerus
Actions—medial rotation (also assists in extension, adduction)

Note: All rotator cuff muscles (supraspinatus, infraspinatus, teres minor, subscapularis) pull the head of the humerus into the glenoid fossa to stabilize and prevent dislocation of the shoulder.

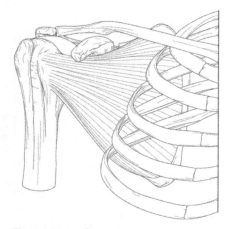

Figure 5.20   Subscapularis muscle.

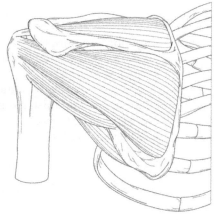

Figure 5.21   Rotator cuff muscles, posterior view.

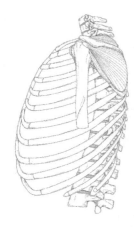

Figure 5.22   Rotator cuff muscles, lateral view.

Assistant Muscles of the Shoulder Joint

Biceps Brachii—(long-and shorthead)—flexion, horizontal flexion, abduction (long), abduction (short)

Triceps Brachii—longhead—extension, horizontal extension, adduction

Summary of Actions at the Shoulder Joint

Flexion

1. Anterior Deltoid
2. Pectoralis Major (clavicular portion)
3. Coracobrachialis
4. Assistants (biceps brachii)

Extension

1. Posterior Deltoid
2. Pectoralis Major (sternal portion)
3. Latissimus Dorsi
4. Teres Major
5. Assistants (subscapularis, infraspinatus, teres minor, longhead of triceps)

Abduction

1. Middle Deltoid
2. Supraspinatus
3. Assistants (anterior deltoid, posterior deltoid, biceps brachii)

Adduction

1. Pectoralis Major (sternal portion)
2. Latissimus Dorsi
3. Teres Major
4. Coracobrachialis
5. Assistants (teres minor, infraspinatus, subscapularis, triceps brachii longhead)

Medial Rotation

1. Pectoralis Major (sternal and clavicular portions)
2. Anterior Deltoid
3. Subscapularis
4. Latissimus Dorsi
5. Teres Major

Lateral Rotation

1. Posterior Deltoid
2. Teres Minor
3. Infraspinatus

Horizontal Flexion

1. Anterior Deltoid
2. Pectoralis Major (sternal and clavicular portion)
3. Coracobrachialis
4. Assistants (subscapularis, biceps brachii)

Horizontal Extension

1. Posterior Deltoid
2. Latissimus Dorsi
3. Teres Major
4. Assistants (teres minor, infraspinatus, triceps brachii longhead)

WORKSHEET 5.1

Muscles of the Shoulder Joint

Muscles	Origin	Insertion	Actions
Pectoralis Major			
Clavicular	_____	_____	flex, med rot, hor flex
Sternal	_____	_____	ext, med rot, hor flex, add
Deltoid			
Anterior	_____	_____	flex, hor flex, med rot
Middle	_____	_____	abduction
Posterior	_____	_____	ext, hor ext, lat rot
Coracobrachialis	_____	_____	flex, hor flex, add
Latissimus Dorsi	_____	_____	ext, add, hor ext, med rot
Teres Major	_____	_____	ext, add, hor ext, med rot
Teres Minor	_____	_____	lateral rotation
Infraspinatus	_____	_____	lateral rotation
Supraspinatus	_____	_____	abduction
Subscapularis	_____	_____	medial rotation

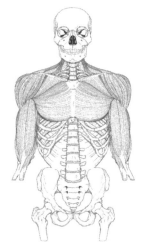

Figure 5.23 Shoulder muscles, anterior view.

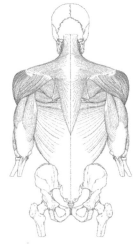

Figure 5.24 Shoulder muscles, posterior view.

Name _____   Lab Section _____

Muscles of the Shoulder Joint

For the following pictures, identify (with arrows) as many muscles as possible that act on the shoulder joint, shoulder girdle, trunk, and neck.

1.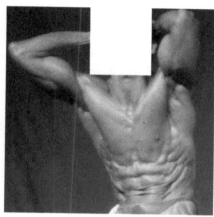

2.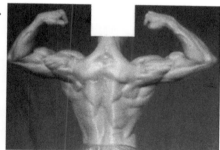

3.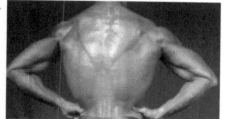

4.

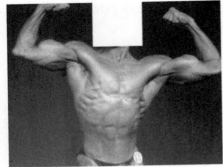

5.

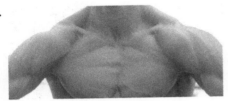

6.

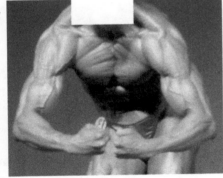

7.

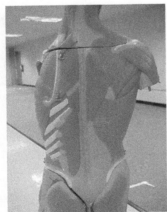

8.

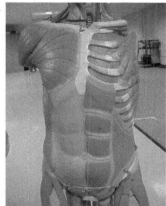

9.

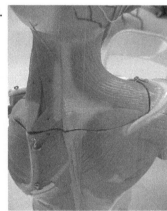

Muscles of the Shoulder Joint

Muscle Action at the Shoulder Joint

1. Abduction of the shoulder
   Shoulder Joint: abduction and possible lateral rotation
   Scapula: upward rotation of the scapula
   Subject: Standing, abduct the shoulder 90 degrees with elbow fully extended. DO NOT elevate the shoulder.
   Assistant: Resist movement by exerting pressure downward on subject's elbow.
   1) Palpate the three portions of the deltoid and tell which parts contract.
   2) Palpate the four parts of the trapezius and tell which parts contract.
   3) Does the pectoralis major contract during any part of the movement? If so, when?
2. Adduction of the shoulder
   Shoulder Joint: adduction and possible medial rotation
   Scapula: downward rotation
   Subject: Standing with shoulder abducted 90 degrees, adduct shoulder 45 degrees.
   Assistant: Resist movement by exerting pressure upward on subject's elbow.
   1) Palpate the latissimus dorsi, pectoralis major, and posterior deltoid.
   2) Do they each contract? If so, when?
3. Flexion of the shoulder
   Shoulder Joint: flexion
   Scapula: upward rotation and probably some abduction/protraction
   Subject: Standing, flex the shoulder 90 degrees with elbow fully extended. DO NOT elevate the shoulder.
   Assistant: Resist movement by exerting pressure downward on the subject's elbow.
   1) Palpate the anterior deltoid and the pectoralis major.
   2) Do both the sternal and clavicular portions of the pectoralis major contract?
   3) Was this what you expected? Why or why not?
4. Extension of the shoulder
   Shoulder: extension
   Scapula: downward rotation and probably some adduction/retraction
   Subject: Standing with shoulder flexed 90 degrees, extend shoulder 45 degrees.
   Assistant: Resist movement by exerting pressure upward on subject's elbow.
   1) Palpate the latissimus dorsi and the pectoralis major.
   2) Do they contract with equal force throughout the movement?
5. Hyperextension of the shoulder
   Shoulder: hyperextension
   Scapula: upward tilt
   Subject: Standing, hyperextend shoulders with elbow fully extended.
   Assistant: Resist movement by exerting pressure downward on the subject's elbow.
   1) Palpate the posterior deltoid and the latissimus dorsi.

6. Horizontal Abduction of the shoulder (from horizontal adduction)

   Shoulder: horizontal abduction and possibly some lateral rotation

   Scapula: adduction/retraction

   Subject: Standing with shoulders flexed 90 degrees and palms down, horizontally abduct the shoulders.

   Assistant: Resist movement by exerting pressure medially on the subject's elbows.

   1) Palpate the posterior deltoid and latissimus dorsi.

   2) What other muscles can be palpated?

7. Horizontal Adduction of the shoulder (from horizontal abduction)

   Shoulder: horizontal abduction and possibly some medial rotation

   Scapula: abduction/protraction

   Subject: Standing with shoulders abducted 90 degrees and palms down, horizontally adduct the shoulders.

   Assistant: Stand behind subject and resist movement by holding the elbows.

   1) Palpate the anterior deltoid and pectoralis major.

   2) How do the actions of these muscles compare to the findings when performing shoulder flexion?

CHAPTER 6

Muscles of the Elbow and Radio-Ulnar Joint

Objectives

To be able to:

1. locate and identify the muscles that act on the elbow and radio-ulnar joint
2. identify the actions of a given muscle at the elbow and radio-ulnar joint
3. identify the muscles of the elbow and radio-ulnar joint involved in a given action or activity
4. identify and locate the origins and insertions of the muscles of the elbow and radio-ulnar joint
5. identify the muscles of the elbow and radio-ulnar joint when given the origins andor insertions
6. determine from the origins and insertions, the muscles action(s) on the elbow and radio-ulnar joint

Muscles of the Elbow and Radio-Ulnar Joint

Biceps Brachii

Origin—(Longhead)—superior margin of glenoid fossa
    —(Shorthead)—coracoid process of scapula
Insertion—radial tuberosity
Actions—Shoulder—assists in flexion, horizontal flexion, abduction
    —Elbow—flexion
    —Radioulnar—supination

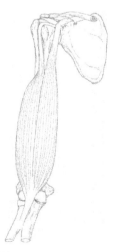

Figure 6.1 Biceps brachii muscle.

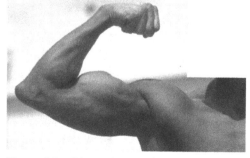

Figure 6.2 Biceps brachii (longhead and shorthead).

123

Brachialis

Origin—distal half of anterior surface of humerus
Insertion—coronoid process of ulna
Actions—elbow flexion

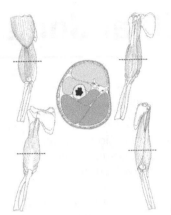

Figure 6.3   Brachium, cross section.

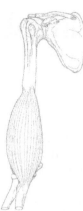

Figure 6.4 Brachialis muscle.

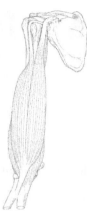

Figure 6.5 Anterior brachial muscles.

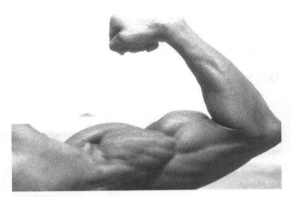

Figure 6.6   Brachialis.

Brachioradialis

Origin—superior two-thirds of lateral epicondyle of humerus
Insertion—styloid process of radius
Actions—Elbow—flexion
        —Radioulnar—pronation from a supinated position to a neutral position
        —supination from a pronated position to a neutral position

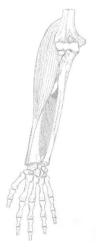

Figure 6.7 Brachioradialis muscle.

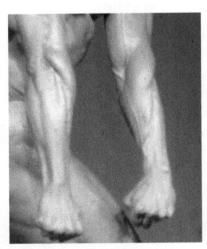

Figure 6.8   Brachioradialis (forearm pronated).

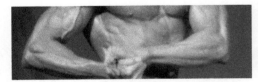

Figure 6.9   Brachioradialis (forearm supinated).

Pronator Teres

Origin—(Humeral head)—superior half of anterior
    surface of the medial epicondyle of humerus
    —(Ulnar head)—medial surface of the
    coronoid process of the ulna
Insertion—middle portion on the lateral side of the
    shaft of radius
Actions—Elbow—flexion
    —Radioulnar—pronation

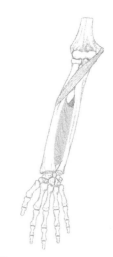

Figure 6.10   Pronator
teres muscle.

Pronator Quadratus

Origin—distal one-fourth of anterior surface of ulna
Insertion—distal one-fourth of anterior surface of
    radius
Actions—pronation of radio-ulnar joint

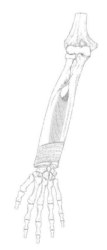

Figure 6.11   Pronator
quadratus muscle.

Triceps Brachii

Origin—(Longhead)—lower edge
    of glenoid fossa of scapula
    —(Lateral head)—superior
    half of lateral posterior
    surface of humerus
    —(Medial head)—inferior
    two-thirds of posterior
    surface of humerus
Insertion—proximal posterior
    surface of olecranon
    process of ulna
Actions—Shoulder—assists in
    extension, adduction,
    and horizontal exten-
    sion for longhead only
    —Elbow—extension

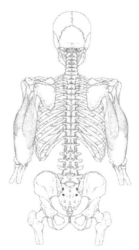

Figure 6.12   Triceps
brachii muscle 1.

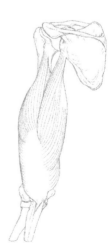

Figure 6.13
Triceps brachii
muscle 2.

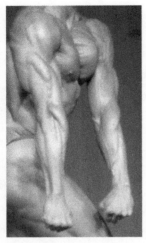

Figure 6.14   Upper limb muscles.

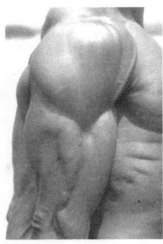

Figure 6.15   Triceps brachii contracted (medial head, long head, lateral head).

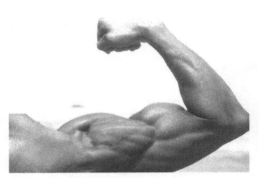

Figure 6.16   Triceps brachii relaxed (medial head, long head, lateral head).

Anconeus

Origin—posterior surface of lateral epicondyle of humerus

Insertion—lateral surface of olecranon process and proximal posterior one-fourth of the lateral surface of ulna

Action—elbow extenison

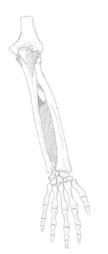

Figure 6.17   Anconeus muscle.

Supinator

Origin—lateral epicondyle of humerus and proximal one-fourth of the lateral surface of ulna

Insertion—lateral surface of proximal one-third of radius

Actions—Elbow—assists in extension
    —Radioulnar—supination

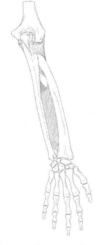

Figure 6.18   Supinator muscle.

Assistant Flexors of the Elbow Joint

1. flexor carpi radialis
2. flexor carpi ulnaris
3. flexor digitorum superficialis (sublimis)
4. palmaris longus

Assistant Extensors of the Elbow Joint

1. extensor carpi ulnaris
2. extensor carpi radialis (longus and brevis)
3. extensor digitorum communis
4. extensor digiti minimi

Summary of Actions at the Elbow and Radio-Ulnar Joint

Elbow Flexion

1. Biceps Brachii
2. Brachialis
3. Brachioradialis
4. Pronator Teres
5. Assistants (flexor carpi radialis, flexor carpi ulnaris, flexor digitorum superficialis, palmaris longus)

Elbow Extension

1. Triceps Brachii
2. Anconeus
3. Assistants (supinator, extensor carpi ulnaris, extensor carpi radialis longus and brevis, extensor digitorum communis, extensor digiti minimi)

Pronation of Radio-ulnar Joint

1. Pronator Teres
2. Pronator Quadratus
3. Brachioradialis (pronation only to a neutral position)

Supination of Radio-ulnar Joint

1. Biceps Brachii
2. Supinator
3. Brachioradialis (supination only to a neutral position)

WORKSHEET 6.1

Muscles of the Elbow and Radio-Ulnar Joint

Muscles	Origin	Insertion	Actions
Biceps Brachii			
Longhead	_____	_____	flexion, supination
Shorthead	_____	_____	flexion, supination
Brachialis	_____	_____	flexion
Brachioradialis	_____	_____	flexion, pronation, supination
Pronator Teres	_____	_____	flexion, pronation
Pronator Quadratus	_____	_____	pronation
Triceps Brachii			
Longhead	_____	_____	extension
Medial head	_____	_____	extension
Lateral head	_____	_____	extension
Anconeus	_____	_____	extension
Supinator	_____	_____	supination

Name _____   Lab Section _____

WORKSHEET 6.2

Muscles of the Elbow and Radio-Ulnar Joint

For the following pictures, identify (with arrows) as many muscles as possible that act on the elbow and radio-ulnar joint.

1.

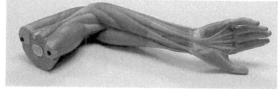

2.

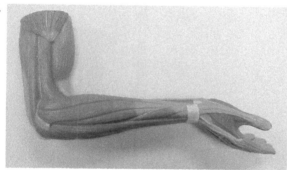

3.

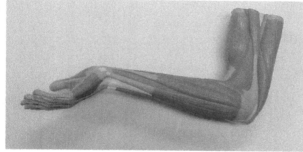

4.

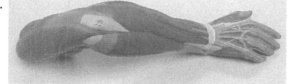

Muscles of the Elbow and Radio-Ulnar Joint

Muscle Action at the Elbow and Radio-Ulnar Joint

1. Flexion of the elbow
   Subject: Sit with entire arm resting on a table. Flex the elbow with the radio-ulnar joint a) fully supinated, b) neutral, and c) fully pronated.
   Assistant: Resist the movements by holding the wrist. Steady the upper arm if necessary.
   1) Palpate as many of the forearm flexors as possible.
   2) Do you notice any difference in the muscular action in a, b, and c?
2. Extension of the elbow
   Subject: From the ground on the hands and knees, flex and extend the elbow in the sagittal plane in a push-up exercise.
   1) Palpate the triceps and anconeus.
   2) Try the push-up with flexion and extension of the elbow in the frontal plane. Do you notice any differences? What might you expect?
3. Supination of the forearm
   Subject: Assume a handshaking position with the assistant and supinate the forearm.
   Assistant: Assume the same position and resist movement.
   1) Palpate and identify the muscles that contract. What is their function?
   2) Can you palpate the prime movers?
4. Pronation of the forearm
   Subject: Assume a handshaking position with the assistant and supinate the forearm.
   Assistant: Assume the same position and resist movement.
   1) Palpate and identify the muscles that contract. What is their function?
   2) Can you palpate the prime movers?

WORKSHEET 6.4

Muscles of the Upper Extremity

Identify the following muscles based on the origin, insertion, and action(s) provided.

Shoulder Joint

1. Origin: lateral border of scapula
   Insertion: intertubecular groove
   Actions: extension, adduction, horizontal extension, medial rotation

   Muscle: _____

2. Origin: clavicle
   Insertion: intertubecular groove
   Actions: flexion, horizontal flexion, medial rotation

   Muscle: _____

3. Origin: coracoid process
   Insertion: mid-medial shalf of humerus
   Actions: flexion, horizontal flexion, adduction

   Muscle: _____

4. Origin: lateral border of scapula
   Insertion: greater tubercle
   Actions: lateral rotation

   Muscle: _____

5. Origin: sternum
   Insertion: intertubecular groove
   Actions: extension, horizontal flexion, medial rotation, adduction

   Muscle: _____

6. Origin: scapular spine
   Insertion: deltoid tuberosity
   Actions: extension, horizontal extension, lateral rotation

   Muscle: _____

7. Origin: iliac crest, spinous processes, ribs, sacrum
   Insertion: intertubecular groove
   Actions: extension, adduction, horizontal extension, medial rotation

   Muscle: _____

8. Origin: infraspinous fossa
   Insertion: greater tubercle
   Actions: lateral rotation

   Muscle: _____

9. Origin: clavicle
   Insertion: deltoid tuberosity
   Actions: flexion, horizontal flexion, medial rotation

   Muscle: _____

10. Origin: supraspinous fossa
    Insertion: greater tubercle
    Actions: abduction

    Muscle: _____

11. Origin: acromion
    Insertion: deltoid tuberosity
    Actions: abduction

    Muscle: _____

12. Origin: subscapular fossa
    Insertion: lesser tubercle
    Actions: medial rotation

    Muscle: _____

Shoulder Girdle (Scapula)

1. Origin: 3rd, 4th, 5th rib
   Insertion: coracoid process
   Actions: abduction, downward rotation, upward tilt, depression, lateral tilt

   Muscle: _____

2. Origin: ligaments of neck
   Insertion: acromion process
   Actions: elevation, upward rotation, adduction, medial tilt

   Muscle: _____

3. Origin: spinous process of 7th cervical and 1st thoracic
   Insertion: medial border of scapula
   Actions: elevation, adduction, downward rotation, medial tilt

   Muscle: _____

4. Origin: spinous process of 7th cervical and thoracic vertebrae 1–3
   Insertion: scapular spine
   Actions: adduction, medial tilt

   Muscle: _____

5. Origin: transverse process of first 4 cervical vertebrae
   Insertion: medial border above scapular spine
   Actions: elevation, downward rotation, lateral flexion and/or rotation of head

   Muscle: _____

6. Origin: spinous process of thoracic vertebrae 4–12
   Insertion: scapular spine
   Actions: depression, upward rotation, adduction, medial tilt

   Muscle: _____

7. Origin: upper 9 ribs
   Insertion: medial border of scapula
   Actions: abduction, upward rotation, lateral tilt

   Muscle: _____

8. Origin: spinous process of thoracic veterbrae 2–5
   Insertion: medial border of scapula
   Actions: elevation, adduction, downward rotation, medial tilt

   Muscle: _____

9. Origin: occipital bone
   Insertion: clavicle
   Actions: elevation, rotation of head to opposite side, extension and hyperextension of head

   Muscle: _____

10. Origin: 1st rib and costal cartilage
    Insertion: clavicle
    Actions: stabilizes acromio-clavicular joint

    Muscle: _____

Elbow and Radio-Ulnar Joint

1. Origin: ulna
   Insertion: radius
   Actions: pronation of radio-ulnar joint

   Muscle: _____

2. Origin: glenoid fossa
   Insertion: radial tuberosity
   Actions: elbow flexion, radio-ulnar supination

   Muscle: _____

3. Origin: lateral epicondyle of humerus
   Insertion: styloid process of radius
   Actions: elbow flexion, pronation and supination of radio-ulnar joint

   Muscle: _____

4. Origin: glenoid fossa
   Insertion: olecranon process
   Actions: elbow extension

   Muscle: _____

5. Origin: anterior surface of humerus
   Insertion: coronoid process of ulna
   Actions: elbow flexion

   Muscle: _____

6. Origin: superior half of lateral posterior surface of humerus
   Insertion: olecranon process
   Actions: elbow extension

   Muscle: _____

7. Origin: lateral epicondyle of humerus
   Insertion: lateral surface of proximal one-third of radius
   Actions: supination

   Muscle: _____

8. Origin: coracoid process
   Insertion: radial tuberosity
   Actions: elbow flexion, radio-ulnar supination

   Muscle: _____

9. Origin: lateral epicondyle of humerus
   Insertion: olecranon process
   Actions: elbow extension

   Muscle: _____

10. Origin: medial epicondyle of humerus, coronoid process of ulna
    Insertion: middle portion of lateral side of shaft of radius
    Actions: elbow flexion, radio-ulnar pronation

    Muscle: _____

11. Origin: inferior two-thirds of posterior surface of humerus
    Insertion: olecranon process
    Actions: elbow extension

    Muscle: _____

CHAPTER 7

Muscles of the Wrist, Fingers, and Thumb

Objectives

To be able to:
1. locate and identify the muscles acting on the wrist, fingers, and thumb
2. identify the actions of a given muscle at the wrist, finger(s), and/or thumb
3. identify the muscles of the wrist, fingers, and/or thumb involved in a given action or activity
4. identify and locate the origins and insertions of the various muscles of the wrist, finger(s), and/or thumb
5. group the various muscles acting on the wrist, fingers, and thumb according to common origins/insertions/actions
6. identify the muscles of the wrist, finger(s), and/or thumb when given the origins and/or insertions
7. determine from the origins and insertions the muscles' action(s) on the wrist, fingers, and thumb

Muscles of the Wrist, Finger(s), and Thumb

Palmaris Longus

Origin—medial epicondyle of humerus
Insertion—transverse carpal ligament, palmar
             aponeurosis
Actions—Elbow—assists in flexion
       —Wrist—flexion

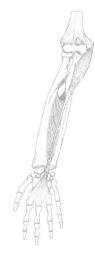

Figure 7.1 Palmaris longus muscle.

Flexor Carpi Radialis

Origin—medial epicondyle of humerus
Insertion—anterior (palmar) surface of base of
2nd and 3rd metacarpal
Actions—Elbow—assists in flexion
—Wrist—flexion, abduction (radial flexion)

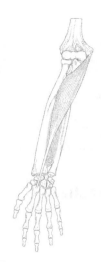

Figure 7.2 Flexor carpi radialis muscle.

Flexor Carpi Ulnaris

Origin—(Humeral head)—medial epicondyle of
humerus
—(Ulnar head)—medial surface of olecra-
non, superior posterior two-thirds of ulna
Insertion—palmar surface of pisiform, hamate,
and base of 5th metacarpal
Actions—Elbow—assists in flexion
—Wrist—flexion, adduction (ulnar flexion)

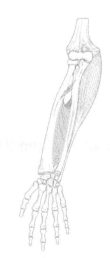

Figure 7.3 Flexor carpi ulnaris muscle.

Flexor Digitorum Superficialis (Sublimis)

Origin—Humeral—medial epicondyle of humerus
—Ulnar—medial aspect of coronoid process
—Radial—anterior surface of middle one-
third of radius
Insertion—palmar surface of middle phalanx of
each finger (digits 2, 3, 4, 5)
Actions—Elbow—assists in flexion
—Wrist—flexion
—Fingers—flexion of MP and proximal
IP joint of digits 2, 3, 4, and 5 (i.e., flex-
ion of proximal and middle phalanx of
each finger)

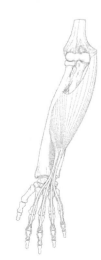

Figure 7.4 Flexor digitorum superficialis muscle.

Flexor Digitorum Profundus

Origin—proximal three-fourths of ulna, medial coronoid process

Insertion—palmar surface of base of distal phalanx of each finger (digits 2, 3, 4, 5)

Actions—Wrist—flexion
—Fingers—flexion of MP, proximal and distal IP joint of digits 2, 3, 4, and 5 (i.e., flexion of distal phalanx of each finger)

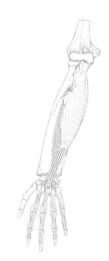

Figure 7.5 Flexor digitorum profundus muscle.

Extensor Carpi Radialis Longus

Origin—lower one-third of lateral supracondylar ridge of humerus and lateral epicondyle of humerus

Insertion—posterior surface of base of 2nd metacarpal

Actions—Elbow—assists in extension
—Wrist—extension, abduction (radial flexion)

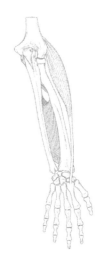

Figure 7.6 Extensor carpi radialis longus muscle.

Extensor Carpi Radialis Brevis

Origin—lateral epicondyle of humerus

Insertion—posterior surface of base of 3rd metacarpal

Actions—Elbow—assists in extension
—Wrist—extension, abduction (radial flexion)

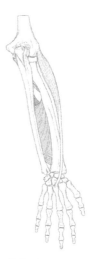

Figure 7.7 Extensor carpi radialis brevis muscle.

Extensor Carpi Ulnaris

Origin—lateral epicondyle of humerus, middle
 one-third of posterior surface of ulna
Insertion—posterior surface of base of 5th
 metacarpal
Actions—Elbow—assists in extension
 —Wrist—extension, adduction
 (ulnar flexion)

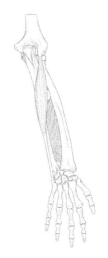

Figure 7.8 Extensor carpi
carpi ulnaris muscle.

Extensor Digitorum Communis

Origin—lateral epicondyle of humerus
Insertion—posterior surface of base of middle
 and distal phalanx of each finger
 (digits 2, 3 ,4, 5)
Actions—Elbow—assists in extension
 —Wrist—extension
 —Fingers—extension of MP, proximal and
 distal IP joint of digits 2, 3, 4, and 5
 (i.e., extension of distal phalanx of each
 finger)

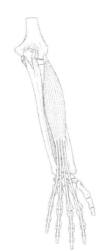

Figure 7.9 Extensor
digitorum muscle.

Extensor Indicis

Origin—distal one-third to one-half of posterior
 surface of ulna
Insertion—blends into tendon of extensor digitorum communis, index finger
Actions—Wrist—assists in extension
 —Finger—extension of index finger at the
 metacarpophalangeal joint

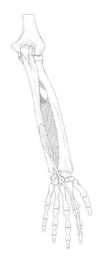

Figure 7.10 Extensor
indicis muscle.

Extensor Digiti Minimi (Quinti)

Origin—extensor digitorum communis tendon
      from lateral epicondyle of humerus

Insertion—dorsal surface of proximal phalanx of
      5th finger via extensor digitorum com-
      munis tendon

Actions—Wrist—assists in extension
      —Finger—extension of 5th finger at the
      metacarpophalangeal joint

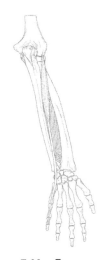

Figure 7.11   Extensor
digiti minimi muscle.

Flexor Pollicis Longus

Origin—middle anterior surface of radius
      (with occasional slips to the medial
      border of ulna)

Insertion—base of distal phalanx of thumb
      (palmar surface)

Actions—Wrist—flexion
      —Thumb—flexion of interphalangeal and
      metacarpophalangeal joint, and adduc-
      tion of 1st metacarpal

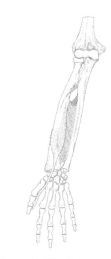

Figure 7.12   Flexor
pollicis longus muscle.

Extensor Pollicis Longus

Origin—middle one-third of posterior surface
      of ulna

Insertion—base of distal phalanx of thumb (dorsal
      surface)

Actions—Wrist—extension, abduction
      (radial flexion)
      —Thumb—extension of interphalangeal
      and metacarpophalangeal joint, abduc-
      tion of 1st metacarpal

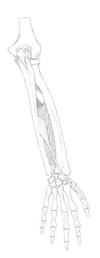

Figure 7.13   Extensor
pollicis longus muscle.

Abductor Pollicis Longus

Origin—middle one-third of posterior surface of
radius and ulna
Insertion—base of 1st metacarpal, lateral
(radial) side
Actions—Wrist—abduction (radial flexion)
—Thumb—abduction of 1st metacarpal

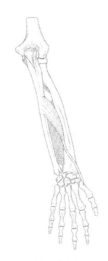

Figure 7.14   Abductor
pollicis longus muscle.

Adductor Pollicis

Origin—Oblique—capitate, trapezoid, base of
2nd and 3rd metacarpal
—Transverse—distal two-thirds of 3rd
metacarpal
Insertion—base of proximal phalanx of thumb,
medial side
Actions—Thumb—adduction of 1st metacarpal

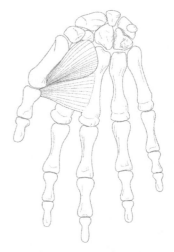

Figure 7.15   Adductor pollicis muscle.

Summary of Actions at the Wrist, Fingers, and Thumb

Wrist Flexion

1. Palmaris Longus
2. Flexor Carpi Radialis
3. Flexor Carpi Ulnaris
4. Flexor Digitorum Superficialis (Sublimis)
5. Flexor Digitorum Profundus
6. Flexor Pollicis Longus

Wrist Extension

1. Extensor Carpi Radialis Longus
2. Extensor Carpi Radialis Brevis
3. Extensor Carpi Ulnaris
4. Extensor Digitorum Communis
5. Extensor Pollicis Longus
6. Assistants (extensor indicis, extensor digiti minimi)

Wrist Abduction (Radial Flexion)

1. Flexor Carpi Radialis
2. Extensor Carpi Radialis Longus
3. Extensor Carpi Radialis Brevis
4. Extensor Pollicis Longus
5. Abductor Pollicis Longus

Wrist Adduction (Ulnar Flexion)

1. Flexor Carpi Ulnaris
2. Extensor Carpi Ulnaris

Finger Flexors

1. Flexor Digitorum Superficialis (Sublimis)
2. Flexor Digitorum Profundus

Finger Extensors

1. Extensor Digitorum Communis
2. Extensor Indicis (extends index finger)
3. Extensor Digiti Minimi (Quinti) (extends 5th finger)

Thumb Flexor

1. Flexor Pollicis Longus

Thumb Extensor

1. Extensor Pollicis Longus

Thumb Abductor

1. Abductor Pollicis Longus

Thumb Adductor

1. Adductor Pollicis

WORKSHEET 7.1

Muscles of the Wrist, Fingers, and Thumb

Muscles	Origin	Insertion	Actions
Palmaris Longus	_____	_____	flex wrist
Flexor Carpi Radialis	_____	_____	flex & abd wrist
Flexor Carpi Ulnari	_____	_____	flex & add wrist
Flex. Dig. Superficiali	_____	_____	flex wrist, flex fingers
Flex. Dig. Profundus	_____	_____	flex wrist, flex fingers
Ext. Carpi Rad. Longus	_____	_____	ext & abd wrist
Ext. Carpi Rad. Brevis	_____	_____	ext & abd wrist
Ext. Carpi Ulnaris	_____	_____	ext & add wrist
Ext. Dig. Communis	_____	_____	ext wrist, ext fingers
Ext. Indicis	_____	_____	ext index finger
Ext. Digiti Minimi	_____	_____	ext little finger
Flex. Pollicis Longus	_____	_____	flex wrist & thumb, add 1st metacarpal
Ext. Pollicis Longus	_____	_____	ext & abd wrist, ext thumb, abd 1st metacarpal
Abd. Pollicis Longus	_____	_____	abd wrist, abd 1st metacarpal
Adductor Pollicis	_____	_____	add 1st metacarpal

Muscles of the Wrist, Fingers, and Thumb

For the following pictures, identify (with arrows) as many muscles as possible.

1.

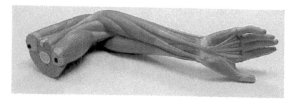

2.

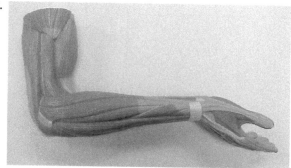

3.

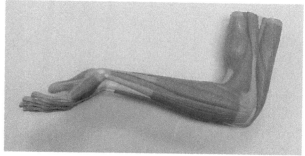

4.

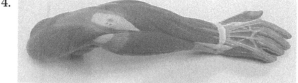

Muscles of the Wrist, Fingers, and Thumb

Muscle Action at the Wrist, Fingers, and Thumb

1. Flexion at the Wrist
   Subject: Sit with forearm resting on a table in a supinated position (palm up) and flex the wrist.
   Assistant: Resist movement by holding the palm.
   1) Palpate, identify, and explain the action of as many muscles as possible.

2. Extension at the Wrist
   Subject: Sit with forearm resting on a table in a pronated position (palm down) and flex the wrist.
   Assistant: Resist movement by holding the dorsal side of the hand.
   1) Palpate, identify, and explain the action of as many muscles as possible.

3. Radial Flexion at the Wrist
   Subject: With forearm resting on a table, ulnar side down, wrist in full extension, and keeping the thumb adducted, raise the hand from the table without moving the forearm.
   Assistant: May give slight resistance to the hand (if necessary).
   1) Palpate, identify, and explain the action of as many muscles as possible.

4. Ulnar Flexion at the Wrist
   Subject: With forearm resting on a table, radial side down, wrist in full extension, and keeping the 5th digit adducted (little finger against the hand), raise the hand from the table without moving the forearm.
   Assistant: May give slight resistance to the hand (if necessary).
   1) Palpate, identify, and explain the action of as many muscles as possible.

5. Finger Flexion
   Subject: With forearm resting on a table in a supinated position (palm up), and fingers fully extended, flex the fingers.
   Assistant: Resist movement by hooking fingers over those of the subject.
   1) Palpate, identify, and explain the action of as many muscles as possible.

6. Finger Extension
   Subject: With forearm resting on a table in a pronated position (palm down), and fingers curled over the edge of the table, extend the fingers.
   Assistant: Resist movement by holding the hand over the subject's fingers.
   1) Palpate, identify, and explain the action of as many muscles as possible.

7. Abduction of the Thumb
   Subject: With the hand on a table where the forearm is in a neutral position, and the thumb is slightly abducted, abduct and extend the carpometacarpal joint by raising it vertically upward.
   Assistant: Give slight resistant to the thumb at the proximal phalanx.
   1) Palpate the abductor pollicis.

CHAPTER 8
Muscles of the Hip and Knee

Objectives

To be able to:
1. locate and identify the muscles that act on the hip and/or knee
2. identify the actions of a given muscle at the hip and/or knee
3. identify the muscles of the hip and/or knee involved in a given action or activity
4. identify and locate the origins and insertions of the various muscles of the hip and/or knee
5. group the various hip and knee muscles according to common origins/insertions/actions
6. identify the muscles of the hip and/or knee when given the origins and/or insertions
7. determine from the origins and insertions the muscles action(s) on the hip and/or knee

Muscles of the Hip and Knee

Psoas Minor

Origin—12th thoracic and 1st lumbar vertebrae
Insertion—pectineal line of pubis and
      ilio-pectineal eminence
Actions—flexion of lumbar region of vertebral
      column

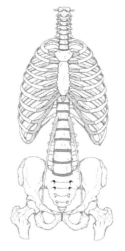

Figure 8.1   Psoas minor muscle.

Psoas Major

Origin—transverse processes of lumber vertebrae (L1–L5), intervertebral
disks of T12 and L1–L5
Insertion—lesser trochanter of femur
Actions—Hip—flexion, lateral rotation
—flexion of lumbar region of vertebral column

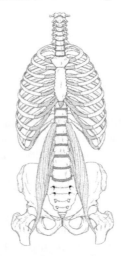

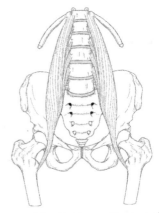

Figure 8.2   Psoas major muscle.   **Figure 8.3**   Psoas major muscle.

Iliacus

Origin—iliac fossa and base of sacrum
Insertion—lesser trochanter of femur and
medial border of shaft just below
the trochanter
Actions—Hip—flexion, lateral rotation

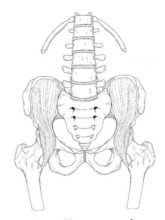

Figure 8.4   Iliacus muscle

Iliopsoas

Iliacus, psoas major, psoas minor
(psoas minor absent in 40% of bodies)

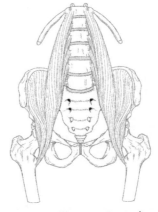

Figure 8.5   Iliopsoas muscle.

Tensor Fasciae Latae

Origin—anterior iliac crest and outer surface of anterior superior iliac spine
Insertion—ilio-tibial band/tract of thigh about one-fourth to one-third of the
    way down between the hip and knee
Actions—Hip—flexion, abduction, medial rotation

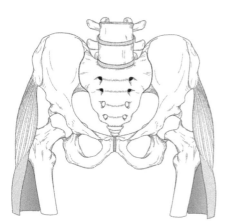

Figure 8.6   Tensor fasciae latae muscle anterior view.

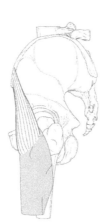

Figure 8.7   Tensor fasciae latae muscle, lateral view.

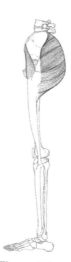

Figure 8.8 Iliotibial band.

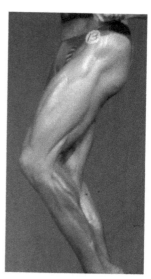

Figure 8.9   Tensor fascia latae.

Sartorius

Origin—anterior superior iliac spine and notch just below it
Insertion—anterior medial surface of tibia just below the medial condyle
Actions—Hip—flexion, lateral rotation
            —Knee—flexion, medial rotation

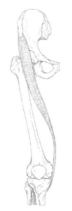

Figure 8.10 Sartorius muscle.

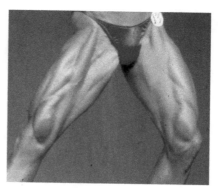

Figure 8.11   Sartorius.

Rectus Femoris (One of the Quadriceps Femoris)

Origin—(Anterior)—anterior inferior
iliac spine
—(Posterior)—superior margin of acetabulum
Insertion—quadriceps tendon to patella, patellar ligament to tibial tuberosity
Actions—Hip—flexion
—Knee—extension

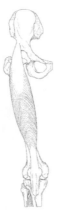

Figure 8.12
Rectus femoris muscle.

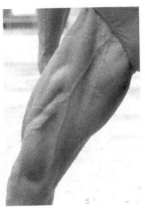

Figure 8.13   Rectus
femoris.

Biceps Femoris (One of the Hamstrings)

Origin—(Longhead)—lateral ischial tuberosity
—(Shorthead)—inferior half of linea aspera
Insertion—lateral condyle of tibia and lateral side of head of fibula
Actions—Hip—(longhead only) extension, hyperextension, lateral rotation,
adduction
—Knee—flexion, lateral rotation

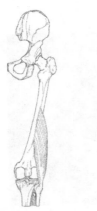

Figure 8.14   Biceps femoris,
shorthead.

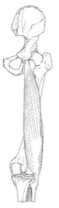

Figure 8.15   Biceps femoris,
longhead.

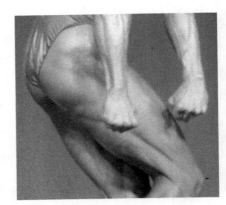

Figure 8.16   Biceps femoris.

Semitendinosus (One of the Hamstrings)

Origin—superior lateral posterior surface of ischial tuberosity
Insertion—anterior medial surface of shaft of tibia just below the condyle
Actions—Hip—extension, hyperextension, medial rotation, adduction
       —Knee—flexion, medial rotation

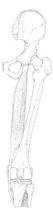

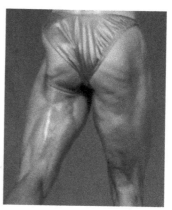

Figure 8.17   Semitendinosus
muscle.

Figure 8.18   Hamstrings.

Semimembranosus (One of the Hamstrings)

Origin—inferior medial posterior surface of ischial tuberosity
Insertion—posterior surface of medial condyle of tibia
Actions—Hip—extension, hyperextension, medial rotation, adduction
       —Knee—flexion, medial rotation

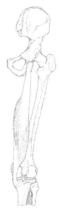

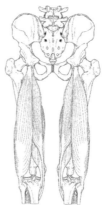

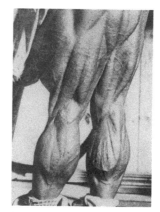

Figure 8.19
Semimembranosus
muscle.

Figure 8.20   Posterior
thigh muscles.

Figure 8.21   Hamstrings—
biceps femoris, semimem-
branosus, semitendinosus.

Gluteus Maximus

Origin—lateral surface of posterior one-fourth of iliac crest, inferior one-third of lateral border of posterior surface of sacrum, lateral surface of coccyx

Insertion—greater trochanter and posterior surface of femur (gluteal line), ilio-tibial band of fascia lata

Actions—Hip—extension, hyperextension, lateral rotation
—(upper fibers assist in abduction; lower fibers assist in adduction)

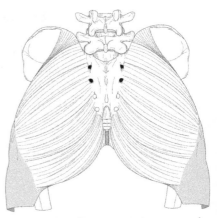

Figure 8.22   Gluteus maximus muscle, posterior view.

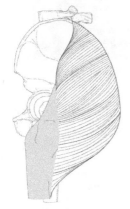

Figure 8.23   Gluteus maximus muscle, lateral view.

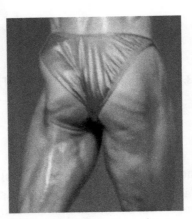

Figure 8.24   Gluteus maximus (relaxed).

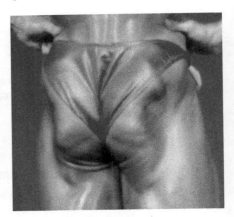

Figure 8.25   Gluteus maximus (contracted).

Gluteus Medius

Origin—lateral surface of ilium below the crest

Insertion—superior, lateral, posterior, and middle surfaces of the greater trochanter of femur

Actions—Hip—abduction
—(anterior fibers)—flexion, medial rotation
—(posterior fibers)—extension, lateral rotation

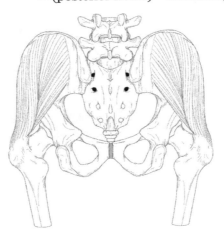

Figure 8.26   Gluteus medius muscle, posterior view.

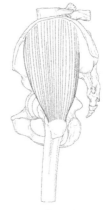

Figure 8.27   Gluteus medius muscle, lateral view.

Gluteus Minimus

Origin—lateral surface of ilium below the origin of gluteus medius
Insertion—anterior surface of the greater trochanter of femur
Actions—Hip—abduction, flexion,
            medial rotation

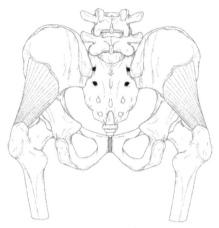

Figure 8.28   Gluteus minimus muscle, posterior view.

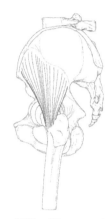

Figure 8.29   Gluteus minimus muscle, lateral view.

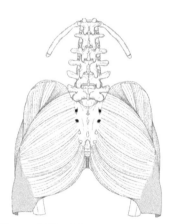

Figure 8.30   Gluteal muscles, posterior view.

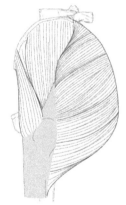

Figure 8.31   Gluteal muscles, lateral view.

Lateral Rotators

1. Piriformis
2. Gemellus Superior
3. Gemellus Inferior
4. Obturator Externus
5. Obturator Internus
6. Quadratus Femoris

Origin—anterior and posterior surfaces of sacrum, posterior portions of ischium, and obturator foramen

Insertion—superior, posterior, and medial surfaces of the greater trochanter of femur

Actions—Hip—lateral rotation and stabilization (horizontal extension if hip is flexed)

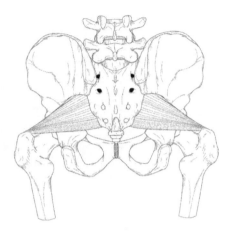

Figure 8.32   Pinformis muscle, posterior view.

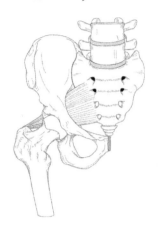

Figure 8.33   Pinformis muscle, anterior view.

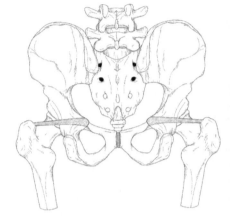

Figure 8.34   Superior gemellus muscle.

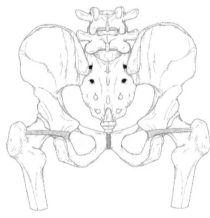

Figure 8.35   Inferior gemellus muscle.

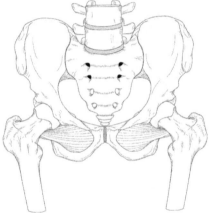

Figure 8.36   Obturator externus muscle.

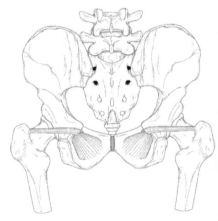

Figure 8.37   Obturator internus muscle.

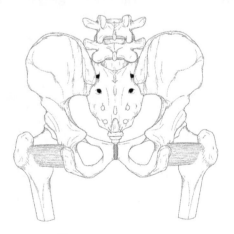

Figure 8.38   Quardratus femoris muscle.

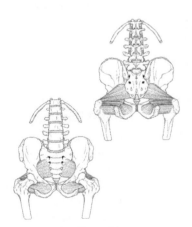

Figure 8.39   Deep hip rotator muscles.

Pectineus

Origin—pectineal line of pubis
(located above superior ramus
of pubis)
Insertion—pectineal line of femur
(line leading from lesser
trochanter to linea aspera)
Actions—Hip—flexion, adduction,
(rotation is controversial)

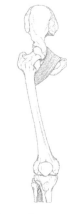 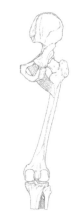

Figure 8.40
Pectineus mus-
cle, anterior view.

Figure 8.41
Pectineus muscle,
posterior view.

Adductor Magnus

Origin—inferior rami of pubis and
ischium and inferior surface
of ischial tuberosity
Insertion—linea aspera, medial
supracondylar ridge
of femur, adductor
tubercle (located just above
medial condyle of femur)
Actions—Hip—adduction,
—(upper fibers)—flexion
(rotation is controversial)
—(lower fibers)—extension
(rotation is controversial)

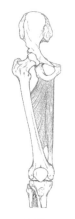 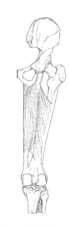

Figure 8.42
Adductor magnus
muscle, anterior
view.

Figure 8.43
Adductor magnus
muscle, posterior
view.

Adductor Longus

Origin—anterior inferior surface of
pubis below the crest
Insertion—middle one-third to one-half
of linea aspera
Actions—Hip—adduction, flexion
(rotation is controversial)

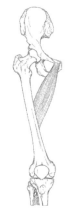 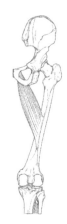

Figure 8.44
Adductor longus
muscle, anterior
view.

Figure 8.45
Adductor longus
muscle, posterior
view.

Adductor Brevis

Origin—inferior ramus of pubis (just below the origin of the adductor longus)

Insertion—pectineal line of femur and upper one-fourth to one-half of linea aspera

Actions—Hip—adduction, flexion (rotation is controversial)

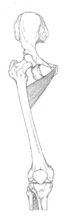

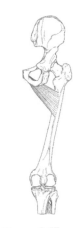

Figure 8.46 Adductor brevis muscle, anterior view.

Figure 8.47 Adductor brevis muscle, posterior view.

Gracilis

Origin—anterior inferior medial half of symphysis pubis and superior half of the inferior ramus of pubis

Insertion—anterior medial surface of the tibia below the condyle of the tibia

Actions—Hip—adduction, medial rotation, flexion (only when the knee is extended)

—Knee—flexion, medial rotation

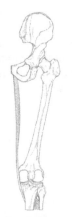

Figure 8.48 Gracilis muscle.

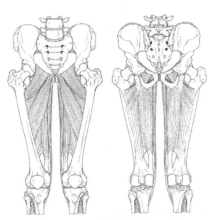

Figure 8.49 Medial thigh muscles.

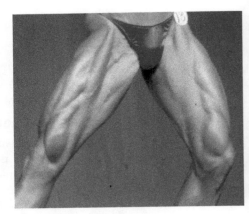

Figure 8.50 Adductors.

Vastus Lateralis (Externus)

Origin—intertrochanteric line, anterior and inferior borders of greater
trochanter, upper one-half of linea aspera

Insertion—upper lateral border of patella and patellar ligament to tibial
tuberosity

Actions—Knee—extension

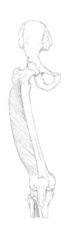

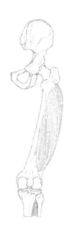

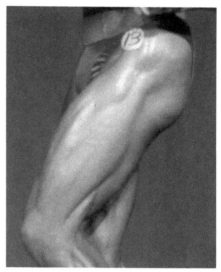

Figure 8.51 Vastus
lateralis muscle, an-
terior view.

Figure 8.52 Vestus
lateralis muscle,
posterior view.

Figure 8.53 Vastus lateralis.

Vastus Medialis (Internus)

Origin—entire length of linea aspera

Insertion—upper medial border of patella and patellar ligament to tibial
tuberosity

Actions—Knee—extension

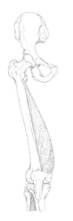

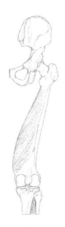

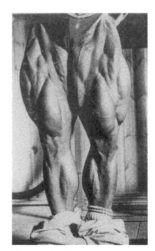

Figure 8.54 Vastus
medialis muscle,
anterior view.

Figure 8.55 Vastus
medialis muscle,
posterior view.

Figure 8.56
Quadriceps femoris.

Vastus Intermedius

Origin—superior two-thirds of anterior and lateral
    surface of shaft of femur

Insertion—superior border of patella and patellar
    ligament to tibial tuberosity

Actions—Knee—extension

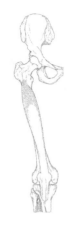

Figure 8.57 Vastus
intermedius muscle.

Quadriceps Femoris

Rectus femoris, vastus lateralis, vastus medialis, vastus intermedius

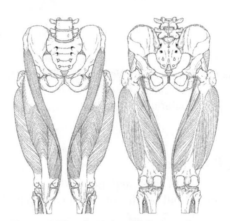

Figure 8.58 Anterior thigh muscle.

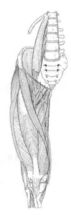

Figure 8.59
Femoral triangle
anatomy, superficial.

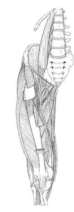

Figure 8.60
Femoral triangle
anatomy, deep.

Popliteus

Origin—posterior surface of lateral condyle of femur

Insertion—superior one-third of posterior medial
    surface of tibia

Actions—Knee—flexion, medial rotation

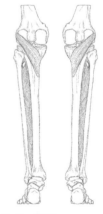

Figure 8.61
Popliteus muscle.

Gastrocnemius

Origin—(Lateral head)—posterior lateral condyle of femur
—(Medial head)—posterior medial condyle of femur
Insertion—posterior surface of calcaneus via the Achilles tendon
Actions—Knee—flexion
—Ankle—plantar flexion

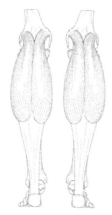

Figure 8.62
Gastrocnemius muscle.

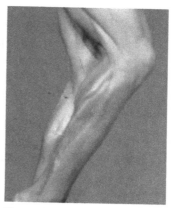

Figure 8.63   Gastrocnemius.

Plantaris

Origin—distal lateral portion of linea aspera of femur
and popliteal ligament
Insertion—posterior surface of calcaneus via the
Achilles tendon
Actions—Knee—flexion
—Ankle—plantar flexion

Stabilization: prevents mov't of femur

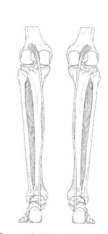

Figure 8.64   Plantaris
muscle.

Summary of Actions at the Hip

Flexion

1. Psoas Major
2. Iliacus
3. Tensor Fasciae Latae
4. Sartorius
5. Rectus Femoris
6. Gluteus Medius (anterior fibers)
7. Gluteus Minimus
8. Pectineus
9. Adductor Magnus (upper fibers)
10. Adductor Longus
11. Adductor Brevis
12. Gracilis (only when knee is extended)

Extension

1. Biceps Femoris (longhead only)
2. Semitendinosus
3. Semimembranosus
4. Gluteus Maximus
5. Gluteus Medius (posterior fibers)
6. Adductor Magnus (lower fibers)

Hyperextension

1. Biceps Femoris (longhead)
2. Semimembranosus
3. Semitendinosus
4. Gluteus Maximus

Abduction

1. Tensor Fasciae Latae
2. Gluteus Medius
3. Gluteus Minimus
4. Assistant (upper fibers of gluteus maximus)

Adduction

1. Biceps Femoris (longhead only)
2. Semitendinosus
3. Semimembranosus
4. Pectineus
5. Adductor Magnus
6. Adductor Longus
7. Adductor Brevis
8. Gracilis
9. Assistant (lower fibers of gluteus maximus)

Medial Rotation

1. Tensor Fasciae Latae
2. Semitendinosus
3. Semimembranosus
4. Gluteus Medius (anterior fibers)
5. Gluteus Minimus
6. Gracilis

Lateral Rotation

1. Psoas Major
2. Iliacus
3. Sartorius
4. Biceps Femoris (longhead only)
5. Gluteus Maximus
6. Gluteus Medius (posterior fibers)
7. Lateral Rotators (Piriformis, Gemellus Superior, Gemellus Inferior, Obturator Externus, Obturator Internus, Quadratus Femoris)

Summary of Actions at the Knee

Flexion

1. Sartorius
2. Biceps Femoris
3. Semitendinosus
4. Semimembranosus
5. Gracilis
6. Popliteus
7. Gastrocnemius
8. Plantaris

Extension

1. Rectus Femoris
2. Vastus Lateralis
3. Vastus Medialis
4. Vastus Intermedius

Medial Rotation (Non-weight Bearing and Knee Flexed)

1. Sartorius
2. Semimembranosus
3. Semitendinosus
4. Gracilis
5. Popliteus

Lateral Rotation (Non-weight Bearing and Knee Flexed)

1. Biceps Femoris

CHAPTER 9

Muscles of the Ankle, Foot, and Toes

Objectives

To be able to:

1. locate and identify the muscles that act on the ankle, foot, and toes
2. identify the actions of a given muscle at the ankle, foot, and toes
3. identify the muscles of the ankle, foot, and toes involved in a given action or activity
4. identify and locate the origins and insertions of the various muscles of the ankle, foot, and toes
5. group the various ankle, foot, and toe muscles according to common origins, insertions, and/or actions
6. identify the muscles of the ankle, foot, and toes when given the origins and/or insertions
7. determine from the origins and insertions the muscles' action(s) on the ankle, foot, and toes

Muscles of the Ankle, Foot, and Toes

Gastrocnemius

Origin—(Lateral head)—posterior lateral condyle
of femur
—(Medial head)—posterior medial condyle
of femur
Insertion—posterior surface of calcaneus via the
Achilles tendon
Actions—Knee—flexion
—Ankle—plantar flexion

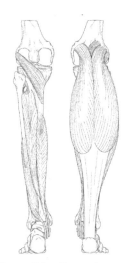

Figure 9.1 Posterior crural muscles.

Plantaris

Origin—distal lateral portion of linea aspera of femur and popliteal ligament
Insertion—posterior surface of calcaneus via the Achilles tendon
Actions—Knee—flexion
—Ankle—plantar flexion

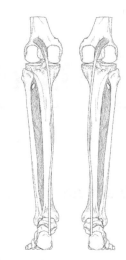

Figure 9.2   Plantaris muscle.

Soleus

Origin—posterior surface of head of fibula and superior one-third of shaft; medial border of middle one-third of tibia
Insertion—posterior surface of calcaneus via the Achilles tendon
Actions—Ankle—plantar flexion

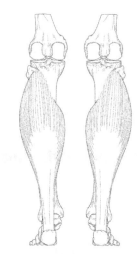

Figure 9.3   Soleus muscle.

Tibialis Posterior

Origin—posterior surface of superior two-thirds of tibia and fibula, posterior surface of interosseous membrane
Insertion—inferior medial surfaces of navicular, cuneiforms, cuboid, and bases of 2nd, 3rd, and 4th metatarsals
Actions—Ankle—plantar flexion
—Foot—supination (adduction, inversion, and plantar flexion)

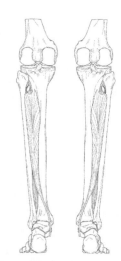

Figure 9.4   Tibialis posterior muscle.

Flexor Digitorum Longus

Origin—posterior surface of middle portion
of tibia

Insertion—inferior (plantar) surface of base of
distal phalanx of the 2nd, 3rd, 4th,
and 5th toes

Actions—Ankle—plantar flexion
—Foot—supination (adduction
inversion, and plantar flexion)
—Toes—flexion of phalanges (2–5)

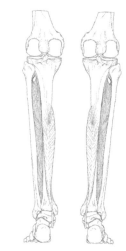

Figure 9.5   Flexor
digitorum longus muscle.

Flexor Hallucis Longus

Origin—inferior two-thirds of posterior surface
of fibula

Insertion—plantar (bottom) surface of base of
distal phalanx of 1st (great) toe

Actions—Ankle—plantar flexion
—Foot—supination (adduction
inversion, and plantar flexion)
—Toe—flexion of 1st (great) toe

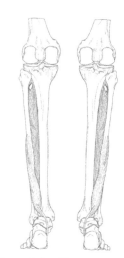

Figure 9.6   Flexor hallucis
muscle.

Tibialis Anterior

Origin—lateral condyle and superior two-thirds
of lateral surface of tibia

Insertion—plantar (bottom) surface of base of
1st metatarsal and medial surface of
1st cuneiform

Actions—Ankle—dorsal flexion
—Foot—supination (adduction
inversion, and plantar flexion)

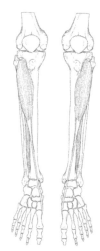

Figure 9.7   Tibialis
anterior muscle.

Extensor Digitorum Longus

Origin—lateral condyle of tibia, head of fibula, superior three-fourths of anterior surface of fibula, interosseus membrane

Insertion—dorsal (top) surfaces of the bases of the middle and distal phalanges of the 2nd, 3rd, 4th, and 5th toes

Actions—Ankle—dorsal flexion
—Foot—pronation (abduction, eversion, and dorsiflexion)
—Toe—extension of middle and distal phalanges of toes 2–5

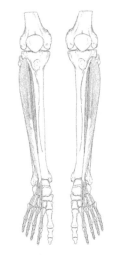

Figure 9.8   Extensor digitorum longus muscle.

Extensor Hallucis Longus

Origin—middle one-third of anterior medial surface of fibula

Insertion—dorsal (top) surface of base of distal phalanx of 1st (great) toe

Actions—Ankle—dorsal flexion
—Foot—supination (adduction, inversion, and plantar flexion)
—Toe—extension of 1st (great) toe

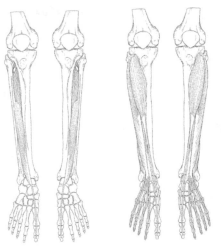

Figure 9.9   Extensor hallucis muscle.   **Figure 9.10**   Anterior crural muscles.

Peroneus Longus

Origin—head and superior two-thirds of lateral surface of fibula

Insertion—plantar (bottom) surface of lateral side of medial cuneiform and base of 1st metatarsal

Actions—Ankle—plantar flexion
—Foot—pronation (abduction, eversion, and dorsiflexion)

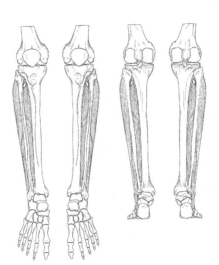

Figure 9.11   Peroneus longus muscle.

Peroneus Brevis

Origin—inferior two-thirds of lateral
    surface of fibula
Insertion—tuberosity on the lateral
    surface of the base of the
    5th metatarsal
Actions—Ankle—plantar flexion
    —Foot—pronation (abduction,
    eversion, and dorsiflexion)

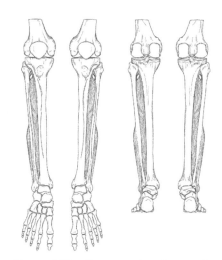

Figure 9.12   Peroneus brevis muscle.

Peroneus Tertius

Origin—anterior surface of inferior one-third of fibula
Insertion—dorsal (top) surface of base of 5th metatarsal
Actions—Ankle—dorsal flexion
    —Foot—pronation (abduction, eversion, and dorsiflexion)

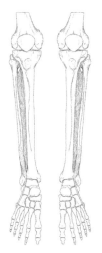

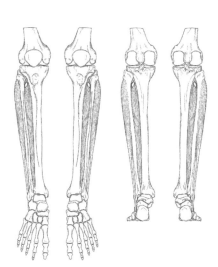

Figure 9.13   Peroneus
tertius muscle.

Figure 9.14   Lateral crural muscles.

Summary of Actions at the Ankle, Foot, and Toes

Plantar Flexion

1. Gastrocnemius
2. Plantaris
3. Soleus
4. Tibialis Posterior
5. Flexor Digitorum Longus
6. Flexor Hallucis Longus
7. Peroneus Longus
8. Peroneus Brevis

Dorsal Flexion

1. Tibialis Anterior
2. Extensor Digitorum Longus
3. Extensor Hallucis Longus
4. Peroneus Tertius

Pronation (Abduction and Eversion)

1. Peroneus Longus
2. Peroneus Brevis
3. Peroneus Tertius
4. Extensor Digitorum Longus

Supination (Adduction and Inversion)

1. Tibialis Anterior
2. Tibialis Posterior
3. Flexor Digitorum Longus
4. Flexor Hallucis Longus
5. Extensor Hallucis Longus

Toe Flexors

1. Flexor Digitorum Longus (phalanges 2–5)
2. Flexor Hallucis Longus (phalanx 1)

Toe Extensors

1. Extensor Digitorum Longus (phalanges 2–5)
2. Extensor Hallucis Longus (phalanx 1)

Muscles of the Ankle, Foot, and Toes

1. Plantarflexion
   Subject: Perform each of the following actions: a) standing toe raise and b) standing with the knee flexed 90, degrees, pointing the toe.
   1) Palpate the gastrocnemius.
   2) Is there any change in the strength of contraction between the different movements? Would you expect any changes? Why or why not?

2. Dorsiflexion
   Subject: Sit on a table with the knees fully extended and the ankles over the edge. From a fully plantarflexed position (as far as your range of motion will allow), dorsiflex the ankle.
   Assistant: Resist the movement by holding the foot.
   1) Identify and palpate the tibialis anterior, peroneus tertius, extensor digitorum longus, and extensor hallucis longus.
   2) Perform the movement with the toes fully flexed as hard as possible. Do you feel any differences? Why or why not?

3. Eversion
   Subject: Sit on a table with the knees fully extended and the ankles over the edge. From anatomical position (plantarflexion/dorsiflexion neutral), try to point the big toe forward and laterally (this can be described as pronation—the combination of eversion and abduction).
   Assistant: Steady the leg at the ankle and resist the movement by holding the foot.
   1) Palpate and identify the muscles that contract.

4. Inversion
   Subject: Sit on a table with the knees fully extended and the ankles over the edge. From anatomical position (plantarflexion/dorsiflexion neutral), try to point the little toe forward and medially (this can be described as supination—the combination of inversion and adduction).
   Assistant: Steady the leg at the ankle and resist the movement by holding the foot.
   1) Palpate and identify the muscles that contract.

PART III

Musculo-Skeletal Mechanics

CHAPTER 10
Analysis of Movement

Objectives

To be able to:
1. identify the different types of work
2. identify the different types of muscle contractions, provide examples, and show applications
3. identify the type of muscle contraction in different phases of an activity
4. identify the phases, joint actions, planes, axes, type of contraction and muscles involved for a given movement

Muscle Work and Type of Contraction

Work (W)

a. Mechanical Work = Force (F) × displacement (d)
b. Physiological Work = energy expenditure (EE)

Work and Type of Contraction

1. Static Work
   a. Isometric Contraction—contraction where the muscle tension can change, but the muscle length remains the same
   b. Co-contraction—contraction where agonistic and antagonistic muscle groups contract simultaneously *(inefficient, uses a lot of energy)*
2. Dynamic Work
   a. Concentric Contraction—shortening of a muscle as it contracts *(up phase of arm*
   b. Eccentric Contraction—lengthening of a muscle as it contracts *down phase curl)* — *muscle soreness*
   c. Isokinetic Contraction—a contraction where the velocity remains the same while the muscle tension can vary *shorten or lengthen at a constant rate*
   d. Isoinertial Contraction—a contraction where a large force is generated at the beginning of the movement to overcome the inertia of the load and generate momentum
   e. Isotonic Contraction—a contraction where the muscle tension remains constant throughout the movement *(muscle length changes)*

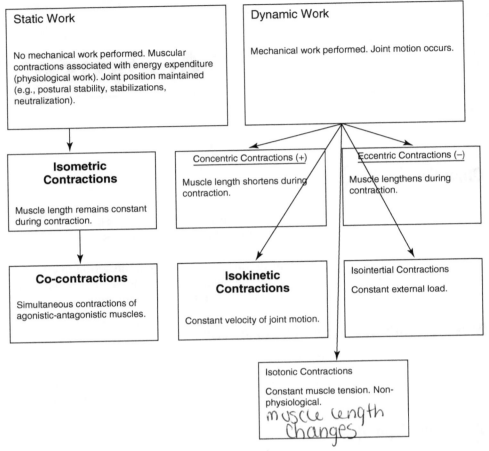

Figure 10.1   Muscle work and types of contraction.

Determination of the Type of Contraction (versus Gravity)

1. Determine the direction of motion relative to gravity.
   a. If the joint action is not parallel to the line of gravity, then it is a CONCENTRIC contraction
   b. If the joint action is parallel to the line of gravity, but in the opposite direction to gravity (i.e., upwards), then it is a CONCENTRIC contraction
2. Determine the speed of motion relative to gravity.
   a. If the joint action is in the same direction as the force of gravity (i.e., downwards) and moving faster than if acted upon by gravity alone, then it is a CONCENTRIC contraction
   b. If the joint action is in the same direction as the force of gravity (i.e., downwards) and moving slower than acted upon by gravity (i.e., controlling it against the force of gravity), then it is an ECCENTRIC contraction

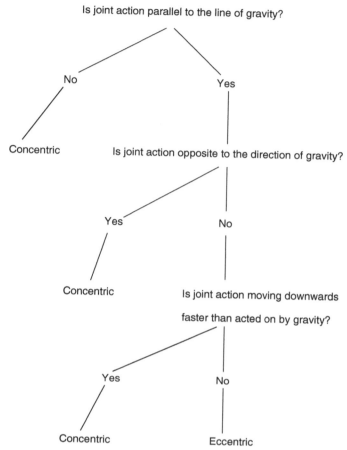

Figure 10.2   Determining concentric or eccentric contraction (free weights).

Table 10.1. Determination of Contraction Type, Muscle Group and Joint Action

Joint Action	+	Muscle Group	=	Type of Contraction
Flexion	+	Flexors	=	Concentric
Flexion	+	Extensors	=	Eccentric
Extension	+	Flexors	=	Eccentric
Extension	+	Extensors	=	Concentric

Joint Action	+	Type of Contraction	=	Muscle Group
Flexion	+	Concentric	=	Flexors
Flexion	+	Eccentric	=	Extensors
Extension	+	Eccentric	=	Flexors
Extension	+	Concentric	=	Extensors

Type of Contraction	+	Muscle Group	=	Joint Action
Concentric	+	Flexors	=	Flexion
Eccentric	+	Extensors	=	Flexion
Eccentric	+	Flexors	=	Extension
Concentric	+	Extensors	=	Extension

Applications of Type of Contraction

1. Isolated movements and contraction type
   a. elbow extension with the shoulder fully flexed or extended
   b. shoulder flexion and extension with changes in hip angle
   c. Knee flexion with the hip flexed 90 degrees or fully extended
2. Controlling the speed of movement
   a. weight lifting
3. Stopping movement of a segment (i.e., absorbing shock)
   a. absorbing shock
   b. for example, landing from a jump/fall, baseball throw
4. Isolated movements, stability, and contraction type
   a. isometric contractions
   b. patterns of ECC-ISO contractions
5. Postural sway and walking (e.g., older populations)
   a. patterns of ECC-ISO-CONC contractions
   b. for example, older populations, pathology
   c. too much sway results in loss of stability (i.e., falls)
6. Sport-related goals
   a. weight training (e.g., abdominal exercises)
   b. kicking, jumping, gait
   c. the ankle (plantarflexion) in sprinting
   d. the hip (angular velocity) in sprinting

Movement Analysis Progression

1. Learn anatomical and movement terminology
2. Develop a reference frame (planes and axes)
3. Provide examples of movement activities that occur in different planes and axes
4. Demonstrate all possible joint actions from anatomical position
5. Demonstrate all possible joint actions in different planes and axes
6. Follow movement instructions given in scientific terminology and identify the plane and axis of different joint movements
7. Provide movement instructions in scientific terminology with corresponding planes and axes to perform a skill or activity
8. Learn to break a movement activity into various phases and sub-phases
9. Identify the joint actions, planes, axes, type of contraction, and muscles involved in different phases and sub-phases of a given movement activity

CHAPTER 11

Muscle Roles and Recruitment

Objectives

To be able to:
1. analyze an isolated joint action and identify all the primary muscles involved
2. identify, for each primary muscle involved in an isolated joint action, all additional actions at that joint
3. determine which muscles are involved, and how they contribute and interact, to result in the desired action in an isolated joint
4. determine which muscles are involved to prevent an undesired action at a single joint

Muscle Roles and Recruitment

Roles of Muscles

1. Agonist—Prime Mover
2. Synergists—Assistants to the agonist
   a. recruited based on intensity and type of movement
3. Antagonists—Act opposite to the agonist (& synergists)
   a. neutralizers
   b. stabilizers
4. Co-contractions
   a. no movement if the opposing torques are equal

Neutralization

Neutralization—eliminates undesired muscle action on the single joint system of interest

Required if . . .
1. any potential *action on the joint* (axis) of the single joint system by an agonist, synergist, or antagonist is *undesired.*
2. any potential *action on the moving segment* of the single joint system by an agonist, synergist, or antagonist is *undesired.*
3. Examples: Isolated movements

Examples of Agonists and Neutralizers Acting on the Scapula

Assumptions:
1. Actions occur at a maximal intensity such that all muscles are expected to contract.
2. Actions are neutralized if any combination of agonist-antagonist action are present, without regard to the number of muscles performing either action. An imbalance of agonistic and antagonistic actions does not imply motion in the direction of the greater number of muscles—factors of muscle force production will do so (as discussed later).

	Upward Rotation		
	Trap II	Trap IV	Serr. Ant.
List All Actions	**Up. Rot.** ~~Adduction~~ ~~Medial tilt~~ ~~Elevation~~	**Up. Rot.** ~~Adduction~~ ~~Medial tilt~~ ~~Depression~~	**Up. Rot.** ~~Adduction~~ ~~Lateral tilt~~ –

All agonists recruited for upward rotation of the scapula will act as neutralizers to eliminate all undesired actions (e.g., trap II and trap IV neutralizing elevation and depression; whereas medial and lateral tilt are neutralized by trap II, III, and serratus anterior).

	Elevation				
	Trap I	Trap II	Rhomboid	Lev. Scap.	Serr. Ant.
List All Actions	**Elevation** – – –	**Elevation** ~~Up. Rot.~~ ~~Medial tilt~~ ~~Adduction~~	**Elevation** ~~Down Rot.~~ ~~Medial tilt~~ ~~Adduction~~	**Elevation** ~~Down. Rot.~~ – –	~~Up. Rot.~~ ~~Lateral tilt~~ ~~Abduction~~

Once all agonists are recruited, the undesired action of adduction (retraction) and medial tilt still occurs. Therefore, an additional muscle (e.g., the serratus anterior) is recruited as a neutralizer only.

	Retraction				
	Trap II	Trap III	Trap IV	Rhomboid	Pec Minor
List All Actions	**Retraction** ~~Elevation~~ ~~Up. Rot.~~	**Retraction** – –	**Retraction** ~~Depression~~ ~~Up. Rot.~~	**Retraction** ~~Elevation~~ ~~Down. Rot.~~	– ~~Depression~~ ~~Down. Rot.~~

If the factors of muscle force production of agonist-antagonist muscles exist such that motion occurs in either direction, it may still be possible to recruit a neutralizer (e.g., the pec minor).

	Depression				
	Pec. Minor	Trap IV	Serr. Ant.	Trap III	~~Rhomboids~~
List All Actions	**Depress.** ~~Down Rot.~~ ~~Lateral tilt~~ ~~Abduction~~	**Depression** ~~Up. Rot.~~ ~~Medial tilt~~ ~~Adduction~~	– ~~Up. Rot.~~ ~~Lateral tilt~~ ~~Abduction~~	– – ~~Medial tilt~~ ~~Adduction~~	~~Elevation~~ ~~Down Rot.~~ ~~Medial tilt~~ ~~Adduction~~

When depressing the scapula, the trapezius, part III, can be recruited if there are imbalances in strength between actions of medial tilt and/or adduction by the trapezius, part IV, with lateral tilt and/or abduction of the serratus anterior and pectoralis minor. Similarly, the rhomboids can be recruited to off-set any imbalances between the upward rotation of the serratus anterior and trapezius (part IV) with the downward rotation of the pectoralis minor. However, when recruiting a neutralizer, it is preferable to exclude muscles with an antagonistic response to the primary action of interest (e.g., the rhomboids) to minimize the energy cost. However, in maximal tasks, efficiency can be often compromised in the recruitment of muscular force.

Stabilization

Stabilization—eliminates undesired bony action—action on any other single joint system (that is not of primary interest)

Required if ...
1. any potential *action on the joint* (axis) *Proximal to* the single joint system (of interest) by an agonist, synergist, or antagonist is *undesired*.
2. any potential *action on the joint* (axis) *Distal to* the single joint system (of interest) by an agonist, synergist, or antagonist is *undesired*.
3. Examples: Isolated movements, complex movements

Stabilization of the Single Joint System—muscular action is to be applied at only one insertion point

1. For a muscle action to pull only one insertion point, the opposite insertion point must be stabilized.
2. This possibility defines the stable and moving segments of the single joint system involved.
3. Question: What muscles act to stabilize the stable segment? Can any other force stabilize the body?

The body, or any part of the body, can be stabilized by:

1. muscle force
2. its own mass
3. an external (environmental) resistance

Stabilization of the Body—if a resultant movement changes the equilibrium of the body (changes in center of gravity)

Examples

The Trunk and the Body

During a push-up, in which the primary action is at the shoulder and elbow, stabilization of the trunk and hips to prevent extension would come from the trunk and hip flexors (e.g., iliopsoas).

In weight lifting, a posture of extreme hyperextension of the trunk is stabilized by the trunk flexors (e.g., rectus abdominus).

Posture and Lifting

Ideal posture would position the center of mass of the upper body directly over the hip joint to minimize energy cost.

When the center of mass of the upper body is not positioned over the hip joint, the weight of the upper body produces a flexor torque at the hip. To maintain a flexed position, extensor muscles at the hip (and the trunk) must contract. As the angle of hip flexion increases, the moment arm length of the weight of the upper body also increases. To stabilize the hip, an increase in the weight's torque requires an increase in effort (i.e., force, energy cost) and an increase in the risk of injury.

Mechanism of Injury in Lifting

The weight (torque) of the upper body places a stress on the mechanical axis of the trunk on the pelvic girdle at L5–S1. Improper lifting techniques can quickly create high risks of injury when shear forces, compressive forces, and joint reaction forces acting at the joint overload the mechanical limits of the joint's supporting structures. Specific pelvic inclinations (e.g., anterior tilt) can chronically produce increased loads on the muscles and joints of the body.

Recruitment Order (in an Experienced Performer)

1. As a general rule, muscles are recruited based on mechanical advantage (MA) and intensity. The MA of a muscle is determined by the muscle's moment arm length.
2. In a submaximal movement, muscles with greatest MA (moment arm length) will perform more work at a lower energy cost and, therefore, will be recruited first.
3. As intensity increases, the need for additional muscular force results in additional muscle recruitment. Additional muscles will be recruited (in an experienced performer) based on a descending MA. For example, the first muscle recruited will have the greatest MA, the second muscle will have the second greatest MA, and so on.
4. At maximal intensity, all muscles (and all muscle fibers) capable of producing the desired action will be recruited. This often occurs to the detriment of isolation of the selected action and at a higher energy cost. However, at maximal intensities, the need for maximal muscle force supercedes all other considerations.*
5. The same considerations regarding muscle recruitment order apply to agonists, neutralizers, and stabilizers. However, oftentimes the need to recruit a neutralizer or stabilizer results in a limitation in the possible number of recruitment options, and/or can produce inefficient movement patterns.*
6. It should be noted that the factors affecting muscle force production (i.e., cross-sectional area, fiber type, and muscle fiber architecture) determine the relative level of intensity and the number of additional muscles required for neutralization and/or stabilization.

*At maximal intensities, it is possible that recruited muscles for a movement at a given joint will produce antagonistic actions (inefficiencies) at other joints upon which they act (e.g., the biceps brachii at the shoulder during a pull-up). At these other joints, the muscle is typically a synergist (i.e., weak actions due to low mechanical advantages) and can be overcome by the agonists at those joints (due to greater mechanical advantage, but at a higher energy cost).

Name _____   Lab Section _____

WORKSHEET 11.1

Determination of Muscle Recruitment for Isolated Movements

Determine the muscles recruited for the following movements at the:

1. Shoulder Joint
    a. flexion
    b. extension
    c. abduction
    d. adduction
    e. medial rotation
    f. lateral rotation

2. Hip Joint
    a. flexion
    b. extension
    c. abduction
    d. adduction
    e. medial rotation
    f. lateral rotation

List All Actions	Shoulder Flexion				

Shoulder Extension				
List All Actions					

Shoulder Abduction				
List All Actions					

Shoulder Adduction				
List All Actions				

Shoulder Medial Rotation				
List All Actions				

Shoulder Lateral Rotaion				
List All Actions				

Hip Flexion				
List All Actions				

Hip Extension				
List All Actions				

Hip Abduction				
List All Actions				

Hip Adduction					
List All Actions					

Hip Medial Rotation					
List All Actions					

	Hip Lateral Rotation				
List All Actions					

CHAPTER 12

Skeletal Mechanics

Objectives

To be able to:
1. identify the different types of machine found in the body and their functions
2. identify the function of levers and the various parts of a lever
3. identify the various lever classifications and provide examples of different levers found in the body and in resistance training machines
4. identify the muscle line of force acting on a lever system, the moment arm length, and mechanical advantage/disadvantage
5. identify the functions of a pulley
6. identify and provide examples of the different pulley classifications in the body
7. explain the purposes, similarities, and differences between pulleys and cams in resistance training machines
8. identify the functions of a wheel and axle and provide examples found in the body
9. identify what combination of levers, pulleys, cams, and/or wheel and axle are used in different types of resistance training machines

Machines

Types of Machines in the Body
1. Lever
2. Pulley
3. Wheel and Axle

Function
Any machine may be described as having one or more of these four functions:

1. To balance two or more forces (e.g., a lever acting as a seesaw/teeter totter)
2. To change the effective direction of the applied force (e.g., a pulley on a resistance training machine)
3. To provide an advantage in force (e.g., wrench versus a screwdriver)
4. To provide an advantage in the range of linear motion and the speed of movement

Mechanical Advantage—refers to an advantage in (motive or muscle) force where the motive force applied is less than the resistive force.

$$\text{Mechanical Advantage (MA)} = \frac{\text{resistive force (R)}}{\text{motive force (F)}}$$

The mechanical advantage can be greater than, equal to, or less than one.

1. If, R = F, then MA = 1.
   a. This means that the motive force (F) required to move the resistance (R) is *equal to* the resistive force.
   b. In this case, there is *no* mechanical "advantage."   *ex. free weights*
2. If, R < F, then MA < 1.
   a. This means that the motive force required to move the resistance is *greater than* the resistance.
   b. This is a mechanical "disadvantage."
3. If, R > F, then MA > 1.
   a. This means that the motive force required to move the resistance is *less than* the resistive force.
   b. This is a mechanical "advantage."

Lever Systems

Lever systems act in **rotational motion.**

Parts of a Lever System

1. Axis (fulcrum)—the point about which the lever system rotates.
2. Lever arms (2)—the physical connections between the axis of rotation and points of force application.
   a. Lever arm associated with the motive force (FA)
   b. Lever arm associated with the resistive force (RA)
3. Point of motive force (F) application—the force that causes motion.
4. Point of resistive force (R) application—the force that inhibits motion.

The muscles and the weight of the moving lever arm produce the motive and resistive forces. Therefore, the points of force application will be the insertion points of a muscle and the center of gravity.

Lever Systems

1. Since lever systems act in rotational motion, the lines of force application (F and R) *can not* pass through the axis of rotation.
2. The rotary movement that any force can produce is dependent on the perpendicular distance between the line of action of that force and the axis—a distance known as the MOMENT ARM LENGTH, LEVER ARM, or TORQUE ARM.
3. Force Moment Arm (FMA)—the perpendicular distance from the axis to the line of action of the motive force.
4. Resistance Moment Arm (RMA)—the perpendicular distance from the axis to the line of action of the resistive force.

The product of the magnitude of a force and its moment arm length is the rotary effect of that force–moment, torque.

The mathematical expression for a lever system in equilibrium is:

$$(F)(FMA) = (R)(RMA)$$

Lever Classifications

First-Class Levers

1. Has its axis at some location between the force point and the resistance point (F-A-R)
2. Performs all four machine functions
   a. balances forces
   b. changes direction of the applied force

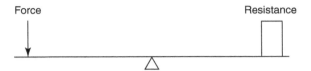

   c. provides an advantage in force

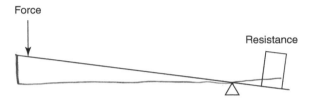

   d. provides an advantage in range of motion and speed of movement

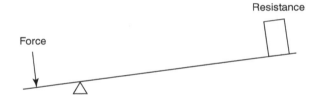

3. Examples—see-saw/teeter totter, crowbar, pliers, a shovel, an oar, scissors
4. Human body examples

Force	Axis	Resistance
gastrocnemius	ankle joint	foot pedal
triceps brachii	elbow joint	weight of the forearm
neck extensors	atlas vertebrae	weight of the head

5. Resistance training machine examples

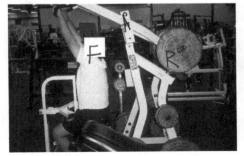

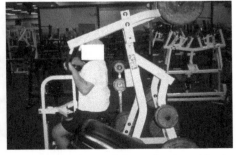

Figure 12.1   Lat-pull down (start position).

Figure 12.2   Lat-pull down (end position).

Second-Class Levers

1. Has resistance point at some location between the force point and the axis (F-R-A)
2. The force arm (FA) is always greater than the resistance arm (RA)
3. Only favors force production

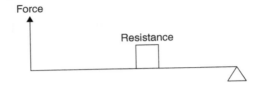

4. Examples—wheelbarrow, nutcracker, a door, a shovel
5. Human body examples

Force	Resistance	Axis
gastrocnemius	body weight	metatarsal-phalangeal joint
brachioradialis	forearm weight	elbow joint
masseter	food	jaw (TMJ)

6. Resistance training machine examples

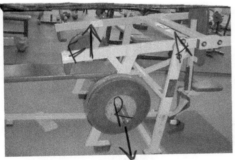

Figure 12.3   Bench press.

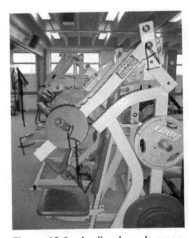

Figure 12.4   Incline bench press.

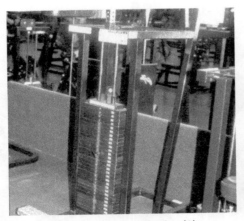

Figure 12.5   Standing calf raise (1).

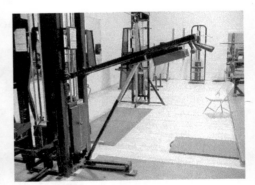

Figure 12.6   Standing calf raise (2).

7. Other example—Push-up.

The total body acts as a second class lever with the motive force applied at the hands, the resistive force of the body's weight acting vertically downward through the center of mass, and the axis of rotation at the foot (i.e., the metatarsal-phalangeal joint).

Third-Class Levers

1. Has its force point at some location between the resistance point and the axis (A-F-R)
2. Resistance arm is always greater than the force arm
3. Provides an advantage in range of motion and speed of movement

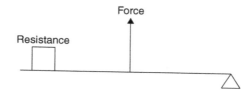

4. Examples—most sports implement (e.g., bats, racquets, etc.), any hand-held object whose center of gravity is distal to the hand, a shovel
5. Human body examples

Axis	Force	Resistance
shoulder joint	deltoid	arm weight
elbow joint	brachialis	forearm weight
wrist joint	wrist flexors	hand weight
hip joint	hip flexors	leg weight

 Most joints in the body are third-class levers. This indicates that the human body is primarily built for mobility and speed as opposed to force.

6. Resistance training machine examples

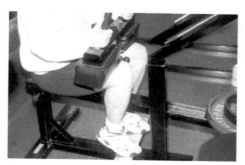

Figure 12.7 Sitting calf raise.

How are these sitting calf machines different?

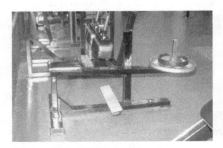

Figure 12.8   Calf machine 1.

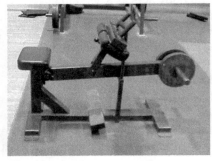

Figure 12.9   Calf machine 2.

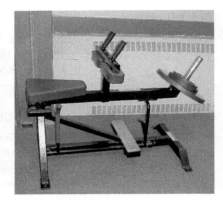

Figure 12.10   Calf machine 3.

How are these rowing machines different?

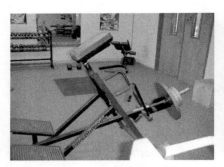

Figure 12.11   Row machine 1.

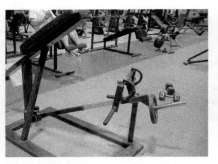

Figure 12.12   Row machine 2.

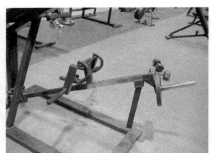

Figure 12.13   Row machine 3.

How are these two rowing exercises different?

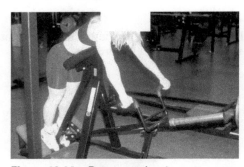

Figure 12.14   Row exercise 1.

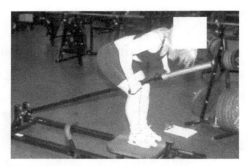

Figure 12.15   Row exercise 2.

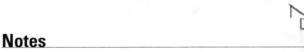

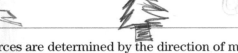

Notes

- Motive and resistive forces are determined by the direction of motion of the lever arm. Therefore, the muscle can either cause the motion (motive force in a third-class lever) or resist the motion (resistive force in a second-class lever).
- All muscles can be mechanically modeled by lines of muscle force acting on a lever system, where each muscle has its own moment arm length and mechanical advantage.
- Note that the moment arm length of a muscle will change with the angular position of the joint.
- In addition, the moment arm length of the weight of the moving segment(s) will change with changes in joint orientation relative to the line of gravity.

Pulleys

Functions

1. Generally, pulleys can be used to create advantages in force, range of motion, or speed of movement.
2. In the human body, the functions of a pulley are
   a. to change the direction of the applied force (no change in the mechanical advantage)
   b. to change the angle of force application (increase the mechanical advantage providing an advantage in torque)

Pulley Classifications

Class 1

An improved angle of pull comes from the muscle tendon passing over an external support. The external support acts as the pulley (e.g., patella).

Class 2

The action of the muscle at the joint is altered because of the pulley (e.g., ocular muscles, peroneus brevis and longus).

Class 3

The joint itself serves as a pulley if the tendon passing over the joint gains a more favorable angle of pull. The joint serves as a pulley.

Class 4

The muscle wraps around the pulley causing the pulley to rotate. By the nature of this pulley, the only action is rotation of the bone upon which the muscle inserts.

Class 5

The muscle acts as its own pulley or uses another muscle as a pulley to improve the angle of pull. As muscle size increases, the angle of pull increases.

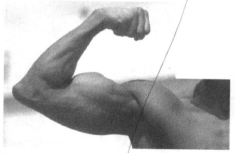
Figure 12.16   Class 5 pulley (anterior view).

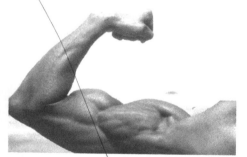
Figure 12.17   Class 5 pulley (posterior view).

Summary

1. Class 1—an external (bony) support acts as a pulley to give an improved angle of force application (angle of pull) (e.g., *patella*).
2. Class 2—the direction of the muscle force at the joint is changed (e.g., action of the superior oblique muscle of the eye at the *trochlea*, action of the peroneus longus vs. the peroneus tertius at the *lateral malleolus*).

3. Class 3—the joint itself serves as the pulley to result in an improved angle of pull (e.g., the *condyles* of the femur and tibia).
4. Class 4—the muscle wraps around the pulley (bone) causing the pulley to rotate and change the direction of the applied force (e.g., the pronator teres around the *radius*).
5. Class 5—the muscle acts as its own pulley or uses another muscle as a pulley to improve the angle of pull (e.g., the biceps brachii and *brachialis*).

Summary Chart

Function	Class
1. Change direction of applied force	2, 4
2. Change angle of pull	1, 3, 5

The purpose of pulleys and cams in resistance training machines are to

1. change the direction of the force/resistance
2. change the angle of the force/resistance
3. provide a mechanical advantage/disadvantage

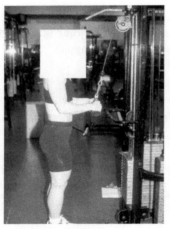

Figure 12.18   Triceps extension (start position).

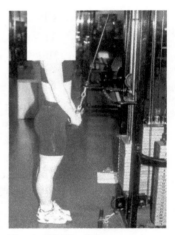

Figure 12.19   Triceps extension (end position).

How are these two arm curl exercises different?

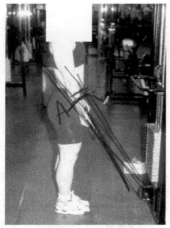

Figure 12.20   Cable machine.

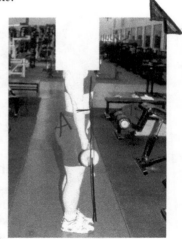

Figure 12.21   Barbell.

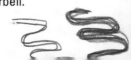

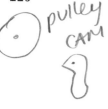

Which of the following two types of pulley systems (single or double) will

1. provide a mechanical advantage in force and why? *double*
2. provide an advantage in speed and range of motion ? Why?

single

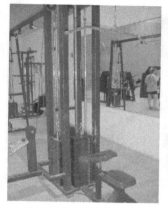

Figure 12.22 Single-pulley cable machine 1.

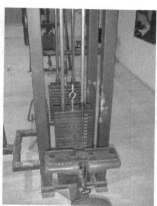

Figure 12.23 Single-pulley cable machine 2.

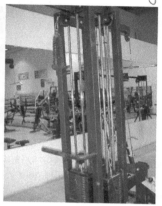

Figure 12.24 Double-pulley cable machine 1.

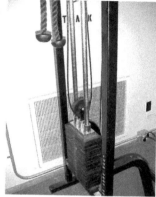

Figure 12.25 Double-pulley cable machine 2.

When cams are used, the force and resistance moment arm lengths will change as the cam rotates (as opposed to the force and resistance moment arm lengths remaining the same when a pulley rotates).

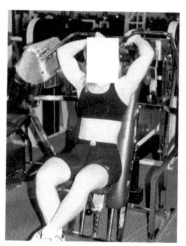

Figure 12.26 Triceps extension using cams (start position).

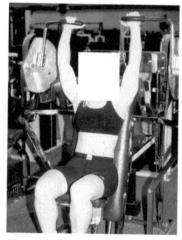

Figure 12.27 Triceps extension using cams (end position).

Wheel and Axle

Functions

1. A wheel and axle can be used to provide a mechanical advantage in force, an increase in speed of movement, and range of linear motion.
2. In the body, a wheel and axle is generally used to increase speed of movement and range of linear motion.

Resistance Training Machines Involving Levers, Pulleys, Cams, and/or Wheel and Axle

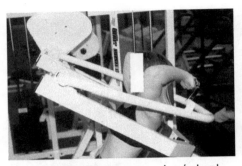

Figure 12.28 Triceps extension (wheel and axle, cam, single pulley).

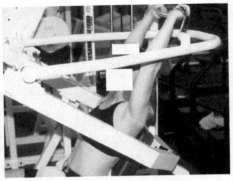

Figure 12.29 Triceps extension (end position).

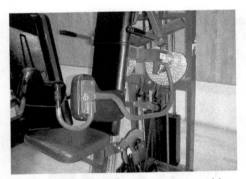

Figure 12.30 Shoulder abduction machine (wheel and axle, cam, double pulley).

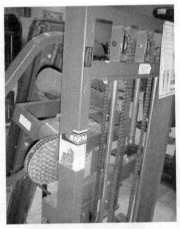

Figure 12.31 Shoulder abduction machine (posterior view 1).

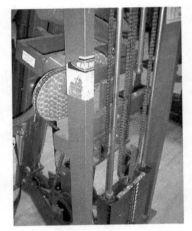

Figure 12.32 Shoulder abduction machine (posterior view 2).

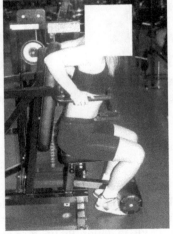

Figure 12.33 Dips (shoulder flexion, elbow extension).

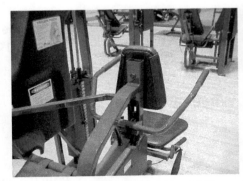

Figure 12.34 Dips machine (back/side view).

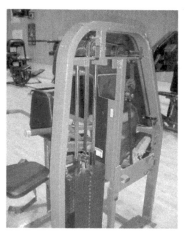

Figure 12.35 Dips—shoulder flexion, elbow extension (cam, reverse double pulley, wheel and axle).

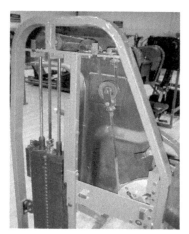

Figure 12.36 Dips—machine (side view).

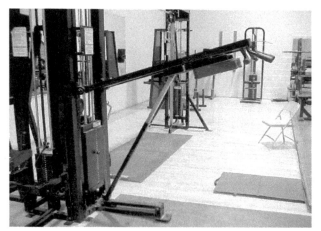

Figure 12.37 Standing calf raise (second-class lever, single pulley).

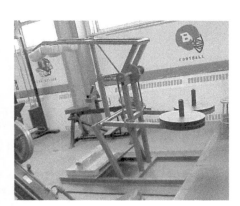

Figure 12.38 Standing calf raise (second-class lever, single pulley, third-class lever).

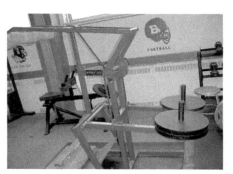

Figure 12.39 Standing calf raise machine (side view).

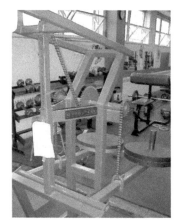

Figure 12.40 Standing calf raise machine (back/side view).

CHAPTER 13

Muscle Mechanics

Objectives

To be able to:

1. identify the components of the musculotendinous unit and explain how they contribute to force production
2. identify the factors that affect force, velocity, and power of a contracting muscle
2. identify and explain the relationship between muscle force/tension, muscle length, velocity of contraction, type of contraction, and power
3. explain what are strength curves and the torque-joint angle relationship
4. identify the factors involved in muscle force and torque production and explain how they affect maximal force and torque production

Muscle Actions	**Joint Structure**	**Muscle Structure**
Configuration of origin and insertion, line of action, number of joints crossed	Degrees of freedom, ranges of motion	Anatomical and physiological cross-sectional areas, fiber types

Contraction Type	**Muscle Mechanics**	**Neuromuscular**
Isometric, concentric, and eccentric. Roles of components of the musculotendinous unit.	Force-length-velocity relationships, power, torque, moment arm length, strength curves. All affected by joint angle changes, muscle length changes.	Activation threshold, All-or-none Principle, amplitude, frequency, summartion, tetanus, frequency-time relationship

Figure 13.1 Factors affecting muscle function.

General Information

Types of Muscles

1. Cardiac
2. Smooth
3. Skeletal
   a. 40–45% of body weight
   b. more than 430 muscles found in pairs (right/left)
   c. most movements use less than 80 muscles

Purpose of the Muscular System

1. To enable the bones to move at the joints
2. To provide strength and protection to the skeleton by distributing loads and absorbing shock

Muscle Properties

1. Extensibility—the ability to be passively stretched
2. Elasticity—the ability to reform after deformation
3. Contractility—the ability to actively shorten

Muscle Structure (From Superficial to Deep)

1. Connective tissue surrounding muscle fibers—epimysium, perimysium, endomysium
2. Within the muscle fiber—sarcolemma, myofibril, sarcomere
3. Within the sacromere—actin and myosin myofilaments (contractile proteins)
4. Forms the theoretical basis of the Sliding Filament (SF) Theory of muscular contraction (also called the Hill Model)

Muscular Contractions

Pathways of Contraction

1. Electrical pathways (e.g., depolarization-repolarization)
2. Chemical pathways (e.g., acetylcholine, Ca2+ diffusion and transport, $ATP \leftrightarrow ADP + Pi$)
3. Energy pathways (e.g., Kreb's cycle, glycolysis)
4. Mechanical pathways (e.g., actin-myosin crossbridge formation)

Factors Affecting Muscle Force Production

1. Cross-sectional Area (CSA)
   a. longitudinal arrangement of myofilaments (SF Theory)
   b. cross-sectional arrangement of myofilaments
2. Fiber Type
   a. Myofilament isoforms determine fiber type
   b. General Classifications of Fiber Type
      • type I (slow twitch, oxidative, red fibers)
      • type II (fast twitch, glycolytic, white fibers)
   c. Mechanical properties
      • contraction (twitch) force
      • contraction time
      • time to one-half relaxation
      • fatigue rate

Mechanical Properties	Slow Twitch (type I)	Fast Twitch (type IIa,IIb)
Contraction Force	↓	↑
Contraction Time	↑	↓
Time to ½ Relaxation	↑	↓
Fatigue Rate	↓	↑

3. Type of Contraction
   a. The type of contraction determines the elastic contribution to muscle force production.
   b. To understand this concept, the muscle can be mechanically modeled as a musculotendinous unit.

The Musculotendinous Unit (MTU)

Mechanical Model

A mechanical model includes only those components that distribute load. During muscular work (contraction), distribution of a load (tension, force) by the musculotendinous unit is managed by the components that comprise the unit.

1. The contractile component (CE) is anatomically represented by the muscle fibers.
   a. The muscle fibers are the only anatomical structures with the property of contractility.
2. The series elastic component (SEC) is anatomically represented by the tendons.
3. The parallel elastic component (PEC) is anatomically represented by the epi-, peri-, and endomysiums.
   a. All of the elastic components (EC) can be modeled like a rubber band.

Type of Contraction and Force Production
1. The force (tension) required in the MTU to create effective movement patterns (speed and direction) is dependent on the load that is moved and the type of contraction used.
2. To create effective movements, force (tension) must be produced in the MTU and applied to the moving segment.
   a. Force production by the CE is considered *active*.
   b. Force production by the SEC and PEC is considered *passive*.
3. When the MTU is contracting and shortening, *all* of the load is distributed (managed) by the CE (the EC shortens like a rubber band).
4. When the MTU is contracting and lengthening, *some* of the load is distributed by the SEC and PEC, and the rest is distributed by the CE.
5. When the muscle is lengthening only (no contraction), all of the load is distributed by the SEC and the PEC.
6. Applications
   a. With a constant load, eccentric contractions are more efficient (require less energy) than concentric contractions. Why?
   b. For a constant energy expenditure, more load can be managed with an eccentric contraction than a concentric contraction. Why?

Parallel and Series Arrangement

1. In the MTU, various components are in:
   a. *series* if they are arranged from end to end (i.e., the tendons and the muscle fiber).
   b. *parallel* if they are arranged side-by-side, or in layers (i.e., the mysiums of muscle).
2. The arrangement of the components of a muscle has an *inverse* effect on force production and the amount of shortening.
3. In a series arrangement:
   a. force production (F_s) is equal to the amount of force that a *single* component can produce.
   b. the amount of shortening (x_s) is equal to the sum of the amount of shortening of *every* component.
4. In a parallel arrangement:
   a. force production (F_p) is equal to the sum of the force that *every* component can produce.
   b. the amount of shortening (x_p) is equal to the amount of shortening of a single component.

$$F_s < F_p \text{ AND } x_s > x_p$$

Muscle Fiber Architecture (Arrangement)

Types (Structure)

1. Longitudinal or Parallel—muscle whose fibers lie parallel to its long axis (e.g., sartorius, rectus abdominis).
2. Fusiform or Spindle-shaped—rounded muscle which tapers at either end (e.g., biceps brachii, brachialis, brachioradialis).
3. Fan-shaped or Triangle or Radiate—flat type of muscle whose fibers radiate from a narrow attachment at one end to a broad attachment at the other (e.g., pectoralis major and minor, gluteus medius and minimus, internal oblique).
4. Penniform—muscle fibers arranged in a feather-like pattern.
   a. Unipennate—muscle fibers extend diagonally from one side of a long tendon (e.g., tibialis posterior, flexor pollicis longus, flexor and extensor digitorum longus, semimembranosus, peroneus tertius).
   b. Bipennate—long central tendon with fibers extending diagonally in pairs from either side of the tendon (e.g., rectus femoris, soleus, vastus medialis and lateralis, flexor hallucis longus).
   c. Multipennate—combination of several bipennate fibers (e.g., deltoid, gluteus maximus, infraspinatus).

Force Production (Function)

1. Muscle force production is proportional to the product of the size and number of fibers (i.e., cross-sectional area).
2. There are two different types of cross-sectional area (CSA):
   a. Anatomical CSA (ACSA)—the CSA of a given muscle at its widest point
   b. Physiological CSA (PCSA)—the CSA of every fiber within a given muscle
3. For a given anatomical cross-sectional area, the fiber arrangement will affect the number of muscle fibers within the same physiological cross-sectional area.
4. Penninform fibers, when compared to longitudinal fibers, with a given anatomical cross-sectional area will have:
   a. greater number of fibers
   b. greater force production potential
   c. smaller range of motion

Muscle-Tendon Length Ratio

1. Penniform muscles generally have short tendons when compared to longitudinal, fusiform, and radiate muscles. In shorter tendons, there is less stretch before the tendon reaches its load-dependent length, which requires less shortening of the penniform muscle. The result of a short tendon is an increased range of motion for a penniform musculotendinous unit. In this case, there is a large muscle-to-tendon length ratio (muscle length/tendon length).

2. As the muscle-to-tendon length ratio of non-pennate muscles decreases, greater shortening of the muscle is required to stretch the tendon to load-dependent length. In this case, the overall shortening of the musculotendinous unit is compromised. On the other hand, a longer tendon allows for a greater potential elastic energy.

Muscular Force Relationships

Force-Length Relationship

1. At less than 50% of resting length, the muscle cannot develop active (contractile) tension.
   a. Passive tension is zero.
2. At normal resting length, the muscle is already in slight passive (elastic) tension. At this length, the muscle produces its greatest active tension.
   a. Total tension is slightly above active tension as the active tension is summed with a slight passive tension.
3. At greater than resting length, active tension decreases and passive tension increases with increasing muscle length.
   a. Total tension is *generally* increasing from its value at resting length. (Note: A 'dip' occurs as active tension decreases more quickly than passive tension forms.)
4. At extreme lengths the active tension developed equals zero, and the total tension is equal to the passive tension.

Examples

1. isolating the heads of the triceps brachii
2. applications to weight lifting (fatigue, 'cheating')
   a. e.g., knee extensions, knee flexions

Force-Velocity Relationship

1. In a concentric contraction (positive direction), speed of contraction decreases as tension increases.
   a. e.g., curling a progressively heavier resistance
   b. Note that the tension developed in a muscle is directly related to the load.
   c. As load increases, required tension increases and speed decreases.
2. With zero load, velocity of contraction reflects the theoretical, maximal, and shortening speed of the contractile component.
3. Maximal force (tension) can be actively produced in an isometric contraction, for which velocity equals zero.
4. In a maximal eccentric contraction (negative direction), actively produced tension (force) is constant (maximal), and total tension increases as passive (elastic) tension develops.
   a. As eccentric loads increase, total tension increases and speed increases.
   b. Therefore, in a maximal eccentric contraction, speed of contraction (i.e. muscle lengthening) increases as tension (load) increases.
   c. This will continue to the point of failure.
   d. e.g., curling a progressively heavier resistance

5. The velocity at which a muscle shortens is affected by the force it must produce to move the load. Therefore, for any given load there is an *optimal* velocity of movement.
   a. The greater the load, the lower the optimal velocity.
   b. An increase in load requires an increase in the number of crossbridges.
   c. If more muscle fibers need to be recruited for a greater load, then more time is needed to form crossbridges.
   d. A greater load requiring a greater number of crossbridges and muscle fibers to be recruited, and greater time to transmit the tension through the series elastic components (tendons), will result in an increase in the latency period (electromechanical delay) prior to the start of the movement.
6. A rapidly contracting muscle generates less force than one contracting more slowly.
   a. The faster the actin and myosin filaments move past each other, the less time available to form crossbridges, and therefore, fewer crossbridges can be formed and less force is produced.
7. Velocities above optimum are uneconomical.
   a. A greater number of crossbridges are formed, but they produce the same force so energy is wasted.
8. Velocities below optimum are uneconomical.
   a. If force is maintained over a longer period of time, more energy is expended for the same amount of shortening.
9. Most individuals will automatically self-select an optimal velocity for a given load. However, the optimal velocity for any given load will vary between:
   a. different activities due to anatomical position (e.g., a wide grip bench press vs. a narrow grip bench press)
   b. different individuals in the same activity due to experience and strength difference (e.g., a stronger person bench pressing a 100-lb. weight)

Force-Velocity-Power Relationship

1. Muscular Power—The product of force and velocity.

   Power = Force $\times$ Velocity [P=(F)(v)].

2. Since velocity is affected by load, power is a function of load.
3. If v = 0 (i.e., an isometric contraction), then P = 0.
4. If force is minimal, power will also be minimal.
5. Finding the highest force that can be developed with the highest velocity (optimization) will generate maximal power.

Force-Length-Velocity Relationship

1. Factors affecting force production of the MTU include:
   a. CSA (CE)
   b. fiber type (CE)
   c. type of contraction (SEC, PEC)
   d. muscle fiber architecture
   e. force-length relationship (CE)
   f. force-velocity relationship (CE, SEC, PEC)
2. Factors affecting velocity of contraction include:
   a. muscle length (the number of sarcomeres in series.)
   b. shortening rate per sarcomere (or per muscle fiber)—this is dependent on fiber type

c. fiber arrangement—multipennate muscles will be relatively shorter and have a slower velocity of shortening

d. the load that will be moved

Theoretical Applications

F-L and F-V relationships may be estimated if sarcomeres behave uniformly. However, . . .

1. not all sarcomeres act at exactly equal lengths (sarcomeres at the ends of fibers being typically shorter that fibers in the middle),
2. not all sarcomeres have identical velocities (remember functional origin and insertions),
3. not all cross-bridges generate the same amount of force (myofilament isoform and fiber type), and
4. only a percentage of cross-bridges may be activated, even during a maximal contraction.

Therefore, the most applied way to describe muscle function is to describe muscle force as a function of joint angle. This is known as a strength curve.

Strength Curves (Torque-Joint Angle Relationship)

1. Strength curves represent *maximal* muscular torque (force) production at specific angular positions of the articulating joint.
   a. During maximal muscle force production, factors of CSA and fiber type are constant.
2. The factors that can directly affect a strength curve include:
   a. muscle length
   b. muscle moment arm length
   c. velocity (speed and direction) of contraction

Factors Affecting Muscle Torque Production

1. Factors of muscle torque production include:
   a. factors affecting force production by the MTU
   b. muscle moment arm length

Skillful Movement Patterns—The resultant speed and direction of segmental movements is the result of the net total of torques acting on each segment (e.g., muscle torque versus load torque).

Appendix

Group Presentation Instructions (40 Points)

Presentation Requirements

1. Each group presentation should be between 10–12 minutes. After the presentation, time (3–5 minutes) should be available for questions.
2. A copy of all materials presented will be submitted to the instructor as a hard copy of the presentation prior to the start of the presentation.
   a. A group's grade will be evaluated *only* from the oral presentation.
3. All group members are expected to be present at the presentation unless acceptable arrangements have been made with the instructor.
4. The order of group presentations in each lab section will be determined randomly. If a student is not present when the group begins, that student will automatically receive a grade of zero.

Presentation Outline

1. Select a specific movement from any movement skill in any area comparing an unskilled/novice/beginner performer to that of a skilled/elite performer.
   a. Excluded movements include weight lifting movements and specific skills presented in class.
   b. Check with the instructor for approval of movement skill selected (since some skill or activity may not be acceptable).
2. A group member or an organized sequence of group members should narrate the presentation.
3. One of the presenters in the group should demonstrate the movement prior to and during the analysis.
   a. Other group members should assist the performer to illustrate key points.
   b. An acceptable alternative is to use video to demonstrate your skill.
   c. All members should actively participate.
4. The movement should be anatomically analyzed according to the principles discussed in lecture, lab, and your textbook.
   a. A completed anatomical analysis must be submitted to the instructor of the skilled performer. *A 25% deduction of the total presentation grade (10 points) will be given without a completed analysis.*
   b. Presentations are expected to illustrate observed joint actions and primary muscles involved in each phase of the movement.
   c. Presentations are expected to compare and discuss what is similar and/or different between an unskilled/novice/beginner performer and a skilled/elite performer.
5. Time should be allotted for questions and answers. Each member of your group should know the movement *completely* and be able to address any questions asked. If the presentation exceeds 15 minutes, no time will be available for a question and answer period.

Grading Criteria (30 points)

1. Time usage
2. Introduction
3. Audio-visual aids used
4. Clarity
5. Logical and systematic analysis
6. Group interaction and active participation of all members
7. Skill demonstration and relevant discussion
8. All anatomical variables included
9. Skilled vs. unskilled comparison
10. Question and answer period

Individual Grades

1. 30 points (75%) of each student's overall grade will be determined by the instructor based solely on the group oral presentation and the grading criteria listed. The instructor will give a group score.
   a. Any student member of a group who is not present at the time of presentation without an excused absence will automatically receive a grade of 0.
2. 10 points (25%) of each student's overall grade will be determined by the members of that student's group based on level of participation and contribution within the group toward the presentation and project.
   a. ALL grades are confidential and should be reported *only* to the instructor on the page provided. Grades should be assigned by each student outside of class. (*Do not* complete the group grade in class.)
   b. Student grades will be submitted (immediately) at the start of the lab period on the presentation day. Any student that does *not* submit grades for their group members will automatically receive a zero for the group grade (25% of the total grade).
3. A self-rating is also included. If your self-rating is within one point (+/−) of the average of your group grade, you will receive one point of extra credit.

Group Presentation Evaluation

Relevant Criteria	Target (3 points)	Satisfactory 1.5 points)	Inadequate (0 points)
1. Time (minutes)	10–12	< 10 or > 12	< 9 or > 15
2. Introduction	topic/presenters/roles	topic/presenter	topic only
3. A-V aids used	3 or more	2	1
4. Clarity	loud & clear, expressive text readable		difficult to hear, monotone text hard to read
5. Analysis	very understandable	somewhat understandable	does not make sense
6. Participation	all	some	one
7. Planes & Views (markers)	3 appropriate ones (correct & visible)	2 (visible)	1 (none)
8. Analysis Chart	complete correct	incomplete semi-correct	incomplete incorrect chart
9. Comparison (skilled vs unskilled)	detailed & complete (clear differences)	brief or incomplete (differences not clear)	brief and incomplete (no observable differences)
10. Q & A	clear, correct response	incomplete, incorrect	can't answer question responses unfocused,

Peer Ratings of Group Project and Presentations

Rate each person in your group on the following items (1=extremely poor; 5=excellent)

Self-Rating (Name): _____

Attendance at group meetings	1	2	3	4	5
Contribution to the class presentation	1	2	3	4	5
Contribution to the written project	1	2	3	4	5
Overall rating of your participation	1	2	3	4	5

Person Being Rated: _____

Attendance at group meetings	1	2	3	4	5
Contribution to the class presentation	1	2	3	4	5
Contribution to the written project	1	2	3	4	5
Overall rating of student's participation	1	2	3	4	5

Person Being Rated: _____

Attendance at group meetings	1	2	3	4	5
Contribution to the class presentation	1	2	3	4	5
Contribution to the written project	1	2	3	4	5
Overall rating of student's participation	1	2	3	4	5

Person Being Rated: _____

Attendance at group meetings	1	2	3	4	5
Contribution to the class presentation	1	2	3	4	5
Contribution to the written project	1	2	3	4	5
Overall rating of student's participation	1	2	3	4	5

Person Being Rated: _____

Attendance at group meetings	1	2	3	4	5
Contribution to the class presentation	1	2	3	4	5
Contribution to the written project	1	2	3	4	5
Overall rating of student's participation	1	2	3	4	5

Anatomical Analysis Chart

Movement Skill: _____ Movement Phase 1) _____ Simultaneous/Sequential/Both

Primary Purpose: _____ Movement Phase 2) _____ Simultaneous/Sequential/Both

Movement Phase 3) _____ Simultaneous/Sequential/Both

Movement Phase 4) _____ Simultaneous/Sequential/Both

Phase 1	Joint (R/L)	Starting Position	Observed Joint Action	Segment Moved	Plane of Motion	Axis of Motion	Type of Contraction	Prime Mover(s)

Phase 2	Joint (R/L)	Starting Position	Observed Joint Action	Segment Moved	Plane of Motion	Axis of Motion	Type of Contraction	Prime Mover(s)

Phase 3	Joint (R/L)	Starting Position	Observed Joint Action	Segment Moved	Plane of Motion	Axis of Motion	Type of Contraction	Prime Mover(s)

Phase 4	Joint (R/L)	Starting Position	Observed Joint Action	Segment Moved	Plane of Motion	Axis of Motion	Type of Contraction	Prime Mover(s)